the Older I Get...

Fern Britton

The Older I Get...

How I repowered my life

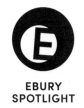

EBURY
SPOTLIGHT

1

Ebury Spotlight, an imprint of Ebury Publishing
Penguin Random House UK
One Embassy Gardens, 8 Viaduct Gdns,
Nine Elms, London SW11 7BW

Ebury Spotlight is part of the Penguin Random House group of companies
whose addresses can be found at global.penguinrandomhouse.com

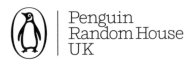

www.penguin.co.uk

A CIP catalogue record for this book is available from the British Library

ISBN 9781529940503

Printed and bound in Great Britain by Clays Ltd, Elcograf S.p.A.

The authorised representative in the EEA is Penguin Random House Ireland,
Morrison Chambers, 32 Nassau Street, Dublin D02 YH68

Penguin Random House is committed to a sustainable future for our
business, our readers and our planet. This book is made from
Forest Stewardship Council® certified paper.

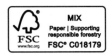

To all women, everywhere. You are great x

Contents

Introduction

repowered; repowering; repowers

transitive verb

to provide again or anew with power

especially: to provide (something, such as a car)

with a new engine

Merriam-Webster Dictionary

*G*etting older is not for the faint-hearted. Reaching 30 or 40, or even 50, is a breeze compared to facing 60. You need time to process the reality of the problem: viz., you don't want to be old.

I am now 67 and often feel the urge to tell people (often complete strangers) my age. Very rewarding when people gasp in astonishment upon hearing this. Not so good when they just nod impassively. Nevertheless, I am still certain that people want to know more about me. I oblige them with 'I've had my right shoulder completely replaced. Want to have a look at the scar?'

What possesses me?

Obviously the need to prove that, old as I am, I am a medical marvel, in peak physical condition, with a tattoo. Young in every way and generally fabulous … for my age. And I want you to feel the same.

If you're anything like me, you're a child of the seventies or eighties who wore power suits with ridiculous shoulder pads. Perhaps you had a bubble perm and went to see David Bowie live and still know all the words to 'Ziggy Stardust' (maybe we met – 1973 Earl's Court). Maybe you flattened a lot of grass with, I hope, unsuitable lovers. And it was fun. So don't pretend to your kids you've never smoked a joint or got drunk.

I didn't expect to write this book, but I've been talking to friends about how approaching my 60th birthday had seemed much more frightening, and needed a lot more processing, than approaching 40 or 50. The trouble is, I DO NOT FEEL OLD. Yes, my knees hurt and I forget everybody's name, but apart from that, I'm fine, honestly. But suddenly it felt like time was beginning to speed up. It made me realise how we don't celebrate enough the joy that can be found ahead. Well, I'm here to show you that a happy future lies in our own hands.

When I had my daughter Winnie, aged 44, I thought to myself that when she's 20 I'll be over the hill, past it, in my dotage. Then, I got to my sixties and, guess what, the sky didn't fall in. Life was the same as it had been the day before. That was a big realisation for me.

So, after I turned 60, I felt a strong desire to enjoy my life and to show my younger friends that it's OK. 'Look, I haven't changed, not overnight.' I had to admit there were cons as well as pros. The main con being I now have a superb moustache and beard, like the sailor on the Player's cigarette packet – but the hair on my underarms and legs has stopped growing.

Anyway, my sixties are ending in better shape than they began.

I was 61 when my mum – beautiful, funny, smart, tough and a goddess in every way – died.

I was 62 when my father, a handsome, funny and talented actor, also died.

At 63, my second marriage, which started the race so well, faded before the expected finish line, and died.

I was lucky in that I could run away to my quiet house in Cornwall, which I had bought many years before as our holiday home. I can't remember what thoughts I had as I got out of the car after that long journey down, but I do remember the house welcoming me, giving me a hug of security and a sense of peace.

There were so many happy memories around every corner. The children dashing in with sandy feet, surfboards piled up outside the front door. The empty packets of crisps and tins of Coke strewn around bedrooms, kitchen and lounge. Happy bronzed and freckled faces of children who were bickering but carefree.

And now, here I was, single, looking at a very different future to the one I had imagined. This was not how it was meant to be. I had always thought that my husband and I would make it our permanent home. A place to share, together, once the children had left school.

Now a new chapter was starting and for the first time in my life I couldn't be sure of what my future held. This wasn't my first experience of rebuilding a life: I'd already been through two marriages, two divorces, two careers – one as a television presenter/journalist, one as a fiction writer. But I *could* do it all over again. I could and *would* create a new sense of belonging and a fresh chapter of my personal history … once I'd taken a few deep breaths and the earth beneath my feet had stopped buckling. Easy peasy. Simple pimple.

Then the pandemic hit.

It wasn't just me who couldn't get organised; the whole world was in a mess. I was lucky that both my daughters and one of my sons were with me. You will remember the glorious warm lockdown spring of 2020? The sun shone daily and those of us who had nothing to do but follow government guidelines spent our days revelling in the silence of zero aeroplanes and traffic. Marvelling at the birdsong we could suddenly hear. It was idyllic and many of us felt the guilt of being free from the harrowing, global news stories of people dying, the NHS at breaking point and doctors and nurses running on empty.

Looking back, it all seems so unreal and I see that although I believed I was handling all my problems perfectly,

I really wasn't. With the distance of four years, I now call it my 'Era of Indolence'. I stopped doing all the things I was used to doing. Writing, keeping fit, getting up with the lark. Even changing my clothes, showering and cleaning my teeth all became things of the past. To this unhealthy mixture I began to add too much wine, too much chocolate and a new hobby … smoking. I took to that like a duck to water.

It took about two years before I could see what it was doing to me and that I didn't like it. I looked old. I grew fat. I was unfit. My knees hurt. Climbing stairs left me breathless. All the energy I had been so proud of – going to the gym, cycling, spinning, swimming, running – had packed its cases and left. I hated my lifestyle and I didn't much like me or my body. Things had to change.

It was around this time that I recalled a conversation with a male friend about fashion. And how women's fashion was all about 'empowerment'. This really irked me and set me thinking. Empowerment? *Clothes* gave women power? Women had no power unless it was gifted by a power suit? The more I thought about it, the more I raged.

The dictionary describes it thus:

empowerment

noun

the granting of power, right and authority
to perform various acts or duties

I don't need a power suit to grant me any of that!

I looked up another variation on the theme:

empower

verb

give someone the power or
authority to do something

Again, I didn't want anyone bestowing power on me, thank you.

Those two words suggested that women had never had any power until it was conferred on them by some third party.

Poppycock and balls to that.

Then a new word popped into my head: Repowering.

I checked my dictionary:

retrofitting and modernising existing power …
restoring it to its original total capacity

Eureka! Something about the word 'Repower' resonated with me. I began ruminating on the truth that of course women are born with power. Just as men are. But somewhere along the line we begin to give our power away. How does that happen? Think about it.

As young girls we were told to sit nicely, speak softly, look pretty. Don't make a fuss, work hard, expect less.

As teenagers, boyfriends hoved into view and we profligately, willingly, wasted our power sitting by the family phone waiting for him to call. Because we thought he loved us? Found us attractive? And because we wanted love. All the complicated emotions. Slowly, and because we hadn't learned not to, we gave our power away. I remember whiling away a whole summer, mooning over a boy who kept me on a string. I didn't understand his mysterious life. The endless things he had to do. Helping out a mate. Working late. Family parties where partners were not included. All the old excuses, which, when they were tearfully (my tears) challenged, were met with 'you expect too much', 'it's not normal' and 'anyway, you're putting your college work before me'. I think in modern parlance this was gaslighting and/or coercive control. The clear message was that we females should just be a bit more malleable and biddable, and a man's life would be much easier.

Then came adulthood and nothing much changed. Women are still too often downtrodden at work and even now we don't get paid the same as men. In 2023, women working full-time could expect to be paid over 14 per cent less than men. We're somehow inured to that but in many ways it's not surprising.

I should say at this point, I have never read a self-help book and I don't think of this as one. I want it to be more like a friend talking, relating experiences and plotting a path forward through life's minefields. I haven't got all the answers, and I don't have a manual. Let's face it, we all work it out as we go along.

But being in my sixties now, I'm realising that, if I want to change my life, it is not the time to sit back in my rocking chair, watching the world pass me by. Instead, it's an opportunity to throw off the layers of characters we have cloaked ourselves in over the decades – e.g. 'sensible', 'hardworking', 'perfect homemaker', 'intellectual', etc. – and to reach back to our younger selves. We knew how to have fun then. We were adventurous and bright and enjoyed life. That 'you' is still in there. Remember her as the old friend she is and introduce yourself. Bring the best bits of her into your future. You may surprise yourself. Whatever our age, this is our time and we shouldn't be afraid to live it in exactly the way we want.

We can find our power, pick it up like a prize and use it.

If you're feeling as if life is passing you by or your world has shrunk a little, if you're missing friends or colleagues and are apprehensive about the future, I have felt that too. Whether you want to start a new business, take up a hobby, find a new lover or just get back some of the verve you had in your teenage years, then you, like me, are a perfect candidate for Repowering.

So let's get on with it …

Look Ahead! The Future Is Fabulous

The night before I turned 60, I searched in Google: 'What can I get over 60?' Here are some of the best things I found, as well as my own list of benefits:

- Once you get to 60, lots of discounts become available to you. Even the Boots card is a thrill as, when you get to a certain age, they give you extra points.
- You have more time to sit and think.
- Holidays get way cheaper once you don't have to go in term time.
- You can get a bus pass – and make sure you choose a fabulous photo of yourself for it. I used an incredibly flattering photograph of me from a magazine shoot!
- Once you hit 60, your prescriptions are free.
- You can watch daytime TV like *Bargain Hunt* and *Homes Under the Hammer* without being judged.
- You don't have so many responsibilities.
- You can get others to do the things you don't want to do, i.e., 'Oh, if only someone could help me with …' It's called weaponised incompetence and I'm all for it!
- You care less about what other people think.
- You're still alive!

Chapter One

When The Sh*t Hits The Fan

*T*here are times in everyone's lives when the sh*t hits the fan. I'm going to tell you about when it happened to me. Don't worry, I'll be brief. The good news is I discovered how enduring the worst of times gave me the energy to survive.

My point is, I had big reasons to Repower and, if I could do it, then so can you. At times we all need reminding that we're a powerhouse, a force to be reckoned with, a whirlwind rather than a deflated windsock. The way I see it is, yes, I might be older than I once was, but really I'm only just getting started. It's too easy to sit around in quiet dissatisfaction, moaning about life and feeling unheard, too tired to change things. But if you want to transform your situation, you are the only one who can make it happen. The turning point for me came when the universe conspired to throw the sh*t at *my* fan. I was without my parents and my marriage and starting afresh.

As we grow older, we expect to lose our parents. It's the natural order. For a lot of us, though, their demise still comes as a visceral shock. The potency of grief and nostalgia is destabilising, leaving parentless people as vulnerable as young children. I remember bleakly thinking, *I'm an orphan now*. But although I'd lost both my parents, somehow, they were still with me. I wouldn't let them go. And it's only now after six years that I've begun to process it properly. I recently had a dream where I was running from room to room around my mum's house, calling for her, but she wasn't there. And when I woke up, I cried. Maybe the first true sign of outward grief I've experienced.

Looking back, I had been dealing with so much when it happened that I hadn't given my grief a chance. Not only was I an orphan, I was also facing being single again at this time. Divorce in itself is a different type of grief and for every person involved there is anguish, pain and a profound sense of failure. I was no different.

I remember going on a first-aid course once and we were given an exercise about what to do at the site of an accident. The first thing was to 'protect the scene' in order to make sure no one else was hurt further. The second thing was to 'assess the damage' of the people who were hurt. Strangely, it's the ones who are screaming that you can generally leave for a moment. It's the ones who are quiet who really need the immediate help. In this situation, I think I was the one who was being quiet and completely in denial, thinking I was totally fine.

In retrospect, I can see I wasn't fine, but I was able to count my blessings and I had many. I had my four children who are all doing well, I had my health and I had a house in Cornwall which has always been my sanctuary. It was somewhere I could convalesce and discover what my new reality would be. Home for me is a place I can be myself, where I can shut the door and withdraw from the world. It doesn't need to be fancy. It doesn't need to be huge. It just needs to offer that indefinable aura of comfort.

I had no idea what the future held, which was pretty scary because I was used to knowing what my life would look like years ahead. I couldn't begin to articulate what was happening to me – but I knew this was something momentous. It was the start of a journey on which I would think seriously about what I wanted at this stage in my life.

I'm not saying I pulled myself up by the bootstraps, gave myself a good talking to and everything was fine. No, no, no. Initially, things went downhill. Fast. The person who used to go to the gym four times a week, did spinning classes, lifted weights and had cycled across the world vanished. I stayed in bed later and later and when I did get up it seemed pointless to put clothes on when I could be back in bed again in a few hours. Other than feeding the cats and making endless cups of tea, I did nothing.

I'd love to tell you a neat story with a beginning, a middle and an end, but life isn't like that. It is not straightforward. When you're going through a tough time you have good days and bad days. Sometimes you get up in the morning ready to tackle the world and by 10am you need to go back to bed because you have nothing else to give.

All of this is perfectly normal. Not much fun, but also not weird. It certainly doesn't mean you're going crazy. Sometimes during a storm there's a moment of calm and, while that doesn't mean everything is back to normal and you're firing on all cylinders again, it does mean things are improving.

If I was going to heal anywhere, I knew it would be Cornwall. I fell in love with Cornwall as a child. Every summer, my mum would drive me, my sister Cherry and my grandmother in my mum's Triumph Herald with her and my grandmother in the front seats, smoking like chimneys. My sister and I would be piled in the back – my teddy bear, Johnson, on my lap – surrounded by the fug of cigarette smoke.

Mum and Nana would chat quietly in the front and my mum's eyes would be trained on the Austin A40 in front, which contained Uncle Paul, my mum's older brother, his wife, Auntie Elsie, and my cousins, Michael and Gerald. Our small convoy would drive – with no motorways in those days, of course – for eight or nine hours, including tea and wee stops. Sometimes, on Dartmoor, a thick fog would be swirling and my mother would tell us stories about the ghostly headless horseman who could appear through the mist. She'd warn us to keep our eyes peeled for him. Thankfully I never did see him, but I was always terrified I might. If that wasn't enough, if we stopped by the side of the road to get out for a break, she would say, 'Don't step into a bog – you'll sink and drown. Oh, and look out for escaped convicts.' Actually, one memorable summer there *were* police checks on the road across Dartmoor because somebody had escaped from Dartmoor Prison. Every car was pulled over and when the police got to us, we were given a quick glance and sent on our way. I remember saying to my mum, 'Why would the police look in *our* car?' And she said, 'It's exactly what a clever prisoner would do if he was on the run. He would disguise himself as a holidaymaker travelling with his family.' For us this was thrilling and we kept watch for him until we were safely off the moors.

From the car, with the vinyl of the seats sticking to the back of our legs, we'd gaze out of the window at the countryside and beyond, craning our necks for a first glimpse of the sea. Having grown up in the landlocked home counties, watching the light bounce off the ocean was more exciting than you can imagine.

We always stayed in Looe, a beautiful fishing town with soft golden sand, where, in my memories, it was always sunny. (It still has excellent fish and chips.) When we finally got to our destination in the cool early evening, I was allowed to skip across the road from our ground-floor holiday apartment onto the shore and run around on the beach by myself. I will always remember the feel of my hot feet on the cool sand, wiggling my toes, burying them deeper into the grains. This was the beginning of my love affair with Cornwall, for sure.

What lay ahead was 14 days of bliss: swimming with my uncle, crab fishing with my cousins, eating 99 ice creams and, most naughtily of all, climbing out the back window of the flat in the hours before anyone had woken up and walking through the narrow passages between the buildings, feeling like a smuggler. I was only six at the time and I knew it was naughty. I only did it a handful of times and no one ever caught me. In fact, you're the first person I've told. Exploring on my own, with no one else present apart from the gulls, it felt like my own magical world, which no one else knew about.

The romance of Cornwall's smuggling history had me in its grip and Looe was a big part of the smugglers' network. Further along the beach, over a stone path known as the Rhyber Pass, were fabulous caves and wonderful rock pools where my sister and I found treasure. I assumed the loot had been left there long ago by smugglers, when in fact my mother had previously gone into a toy shop and bought shiny plastic rings. She'd plopped them in the rock pool, along with thruppenny bits, and we'd spend hours searching, as the sun warmed our upturned bottoms, like ducks dabbling for food. And she'd always caution us to look out for the periscopes of submarines (looking back this was a chance to give her some peace), so we would gaze out to sea, watching as the sunrays glanced off the crests of wavelets, then rush in to submerge our toes.

In those days, a Punch and Judy man plied his trade on the beach. All the children would follow him as he walked on stilts along the sand. After we'd cheered, booed and laughed through his show, my uncle (depending on the tide) would hire a little chug-chug motorboat and we'd trail mackerel lines off the back, sometimes catching supper. That all sounds very Cornish, but what brought a touch of the Italian Riviera to the place was two speedboats, which would take you out for a 15-minute thrilling ride over the water. I loved those boats and I still do. That's when I decided I was going to be a speedboat driver. In fact, I did a course not long ago (which I'll tell you all about later), after I'd passed my motorbike exam, but that's a whole other story. You see, the adventures don't have to come to an end just because we grow up.

Like all childhoods, my own had good and bad bits and, like most parents, I consciously or subconsciously tried to recreate those happy times with my own children. I would take them to Looe every summer and we'd sit on the harbour quay armed with crab lines and a chunk of bacon. I'd use the clock tower as a stopwatch; pointing to it, I'd tell the children we would stay for precisely one hour. Once that 60 minutes of dogged effort and squealing surprises had ticked past, each of the children would count the crabs in their buckets, awarding themselves bragging rights for the biggest, the smallest and the fastest, before carefully returning the weary creatures to the water. Whenever possible, we still go there today and set out our crab lines again – but now they're adults, the competition is much fiercer!

From 1998, we rented a clifftop static caravan on the north coast in a campsite that had pretty gardens, a small shop and a launderette, where I spent a lot of time feeding 20p coins into the drier. There was a path straight down to the beach, so it was holiday heaven. After three years of hiring, I decided to buy my own secondhand static caravan, which meant we were free to come down any time in the school holidays. This felt the very essence of luxury. The caravan was two rows back from those best placed for an unhindered view of the horizon, but nonetheless we enjoyed a great spot. The minute we got there and put the key in the door we felt like we were home. The caravan had a gas fire, a television, a full-sized oven and a fridge. We lived there every summer for six weeks with no shoes on, just running around having fun.

Caravan life is hilarious and comes with its own specific experiences you never get anywhere else. I learned not to open the caravan door too early in the morning because it would attract a flock of children, heralded by a squeal of bicycle brakes. The bikes would be dropped onto the grass outside before the kids crowded into the caravan. I'd be in my pyjamas making a cup of tea while up to eight kids were hauling my children out of their beds. I'd serve them all a bag of crisps and a glass of milk and get them settled to watch something on television. Then, a bit later, I'd look up and they would have swooped off like gulls, as suddenly as they had arrived.

The children still talk about those times today. I hope that I've been able to give them something that they'll look back on fondly their whole lives.

Nostalgia, though, isn't just about the lovely warm glow we get from looking back at a happy time. Used properly, it can be a useful tool for life, too. We can glean wisdom from the past to fuel us for the future.

After childhood come the tumultuous teens. Our teenage years form a chapter in our lives marked by the first real stirrings of self-awareness, the forging of our identity and the pursuit of independence. There's a lot we can take from that as we look to Repower. Teenage years are a time of exploration and self-discovery where we test our limits, join clubs, play sports and immerse ourselves in pastimes that ignite our passions. Memories of those times can be used to drive our curiosity once more, allowing us to feel again that unbridled enthusiasm for life that so often gets crushed under the weight of adulthood and advancing years.

Adolescence is a time of profound transformation and growth. We need a bit of that at every stage of our lives. Many of us don't feel any different to how we did back then.

We're still 18ish in our heads. (Depending on the day, I veer somewhere between 17 and 34.) Anyway, the point is that channelling our younger self has a lot to offer. I think most of us take on new personas with each stage of our lives, whether it's training for our first job, a significant relationship, becoming a wife, becoming a mum or getting a big promotion. With each change we step into a new phase of life and shed some of the identity of the person we were before. I'm learning that we might feel most content when we welcome back all those pieces of who we were.

I was a teenager in the 1970s, which was possibly the best time ever to grow up. The music was magnificent and the fashion was fantastic. We loved Gilbert O'Sullivan, Mud and David Cassidy and we wore Pepe jeans, wedge-heeled clogs and had very short hair. I still can't walk past a fairground without being instantly transported back to that era. I remember so vividly when the fair would arrive on Gold Hill Common in Buckinghamshire, where I grew up. The smell of the generator and candy floss takes me right back to the cool boys, with oil-black fingers, all looking a bit like David Essex – who would jump on the back of the dodgems or spin you around on the Waltzers, while we shrieked to the soundtrack of 'Get It On' by T-Rex, 'Ballroom Blitz' by Sweet or, of course, 'Lamplight' by David Essex himself.

The inky darkness lying somewhere beyond the pulsating music and the flashing lights – it was all so exhilarating. It was one of the cheapest, best nights you could have.

Back then, my friends and I would spend days discussing what we'd wear to the fair. One time, I wore crushed velvet hotpants with American tan tights, because I wanted my legs to look nice, and those wet-look plastic boots that you were endlessly pulling up because the elastic top that held them up would stretch. All clothes back then were either too tight or went baggy very quickly because the stretchy material spandex (did you know it's an anagram of 'expands'?) was still in its infancy. I topped off the outfit with a long, rust-coloured cardigan and felt like the Queen of Sheba, or her rural Buckinghamshire equivalent.

The anticipation when getting ready for such a pivotal night in the calendar was enormous. In my teenage years, the magic for me was all about make-up. I had a black box containing Biba eyeshadows in every colour you could imagine. They were creamy, so within seconds they creased and went all down your face, but that didn't seem to matter at all. In my teens, I was hugely into glam rock and anything with metallic sparkle. I still have a black satin jacket from back then with Lurex lapels.

I still treasure those clothes today. In the garage I have three trunks. The type I imagine children at boarding school would have. I bought them from John Lewis some years ago with the express purpose of collecting my 'History Clothes' in one place rather than scattered about in various bags stashed in the loft. (n.b. Never put anything in the loft if you want to see it again – see Chapter 13.)

History Clothes are those with which you shared the most memorable moments of your life. Mine include a lime-green satin zip-up skintight jacket from Biba c. 1974, a wicked red 1950s-inspired halter-neck dress that got me my first job out of drama school and a pair of tartan trews from Miss Selfridge which I wore for my first television audition. I got that job, too. Oh, and have I mentioned one pair of electric-blue, and one pair of jet-black, spandex cigarette pants à la Olivia Newton-John in *Grease*? My daughter Winnie wore the black ones not long ago and declared, 'Mum, you were so cool.' (I thought, *I'm still cool actually. It's just that other people haven't necessarily realised that.*)

My kids were always saying, 'Mother, stop dancing.' And, 'Don't sing, Mum.' Well, we shouldn't stop. There are millions of us who want to dance to 'Tiger Feet' and I'll tell you something: if I could fit into those black stretchy trousers now I'd still be wearing them. Maybe only to the supermarket, though, as no one has yet invented a disco that opens at 3pm and closes just in time for me to get home for supper. Perhaps we should?

Back then we didn't have TikTok, Instagram or Facebook, but once a week we got *Jackie* magazine. It was our manual to get through our teens. The problem pages were marvellous. Particularly Cathy and Claire, *Jackie*'s agony aunts, for whom no problem was too big. It was their answers that taught us how to practise kissing, that it was perfectly normal to have one boob bigger than the other and perhaps not best to lose your virginity right before your O-levels. How I miss its sage advice.

When I was 17, I met my first proper boyfriend on a blind date. It was so romantic. He was a bit older and had a Triumph Vitesse soft top (look it up). It was a very sexy car. I remember one summer day, between Lower and Upper Sixth, when he whisked me away to the River Chess near Chenies in Buckinghamshire and we embarked on a dreamy day out. We walked in the fields and he'd brought a picnic with a bottle of champagne.

He's happily married now and has children, but a few months ago he rang me while he was having a boozy lunch with another old friend from those days. Both now in their sixties, they decided to ring me up out of the blue to reminisce in the way only people who have known each other in their teens can. Immediately, the shared memories transported me back in time. All the recollections were rather lovely. Here they were, two successful men, loosened by a bottle of wine (or two), returning to their time as exciting, funny and gorgeous young guys. And they transferred that feeling to me. I was buoyant for a good couple of hours after. Why? I think because all three of us had shed the layers of respectability and professional façade that we all wear every day, suffocating our younger, sillier but possibly happier selves. And that is Repowering at its most potent. Hard to bottle but we can try.

What I'm saying is that girl – the one who loved fair-ground rides, got excited over make-up and listened to Radio Caroline under the bedsheets – is still in me. I want life to have as much colour as it did back then. Most of us start life inherently creative and playful and with a real sense of the absurd. It's that fun we need to rekindle. I believe that the minute you stop, life goes rapidly downhill. You lose your spark. Using your imagination is so important because there's all that wonderful stuff inside you that doesn't come from anyone else. It is uniquely yours.

When we're younger, we don't have that fear of failure so much; we haven't experienced the pitfalls of life or the wisdom and understanding of where things can go wrong. We can't return to that time, nor should we, but looking back and remembering the courage of our former self can propel us to discover who we truly are, shedding that façade we put on over time.

It's why – all these years later – I know in my heart that I am in the right place to find my next chapter. Although the journey has at times been difficult, finding the place I belong has given me a solid foundation on which to build a life in where I have the power to be the very best version of me …

Strive for Five

I've got five questions about the teenage you:

- What was your favourite band?
- Who was your biggest crush?
- What did you wear?
- Where did you shop?
- Can you remember one moment from the tumultuous time when you felt comfortable in your skin? Try to recall where you were, who you were with and what you were doing in as much detail as possible.

Recall those times and paint them in vivid colours, so you can be at one again with the fire and energy that characterised you then.

Chapter Two

Keeping the Faith

*I*n life, you must have faith in yourself and trust in others, but sometimes that trust can be broken. Honesty for me is key. When I was little there was a big secret that was kept from me. My childhood was loving, but no one ever told me why my father, the actor Tony Britton, wasn't part of it. If I ever asked where he was, I was given excuses that in childhood I accepted entirely. I knew there was something odd about the circumstances of my birth, but I couldn't pinpoint what.

Growing up in the fifties and sixties, it was rare for parents not to be together. I didn't know anyone else who didn't have a dad at home. My mum was mother and father to me and my older sister. We also had my lovely Uncle Paul and Auntie Elsie, Nana and two cousins, Gerald and Michael. So I had a lot of close family around, but I didn't realise until much later how hard the lack of a dad had hit me. Even today I often find myself wondering what I missed.

When I was growing up, he was a glamorous but elusive figure. He visited maybe twice a year, pulling up in a swish car loaded with presents. Before he arrived, the atmosphere would be trembling with something I didn't understand. Thinking back now, it was high emotion. Expectancy. And on his departure a sense of loss. Anger. Disappointment.

It transpired that my father had left us for another woman when my sister was around eight. As a child, I had no idea where he lived. I didn't even think about it when I was small. What power did a little girl have? I had no address or phone number for him. I think my mum wanted to protect me and/or hurt him by not letting him see me. But that's all conjecture. By the time I was nine, my stepfather arrived and life changed very quickly. I was very unhappy and desperate to contact my father, to ask him to come home. But who could I approach to find out his address? I didn't want to upset my mum or for my stepfather to find out that I didn't like him much.

In the meantime, my father was building a terrific career. As a young child, watching him on television was always exciting and I would wave at him, fully understanding that he wasn't able to wave back because, although he could see me, he was working. When I was about ten years old, my mother and stepfather took me to see my father in the musical *My Fair Lady*, in which he starred as Professor Higgins. After the show, we went to visit him in his dressing room and he took my hand and walked me onto the stage. I will never forget walking out and seeing all the empty seats and feeling the warmth of the audience that had been there minutes before. My father guided me all round the set and the props and I remember thinking, *I want to work in this.* It opened something in me, a possibility.

We didn't see each other often, but he would write letters. I've still got three or four amusing ones he wrote to me. Even though he didn't know much about me or what my life was like, they were always affectionate and witty. Later, when I was 17 and I hadn't seen my father for some time, I decided to take matters into my own hands. I knew my father was staring in a play in London called *The Dame of Sark*, so I asked my English teacher Mrs Calf to organise a school trip for us to see it. Which she did! I still didn't know my father's phone number, so I rather cleverly phoned directory enquiries and asked for the number of the stage door at the theatre. Within minutes he was on the phone, excited to hear the news that I was coming to see the play. I felt a mixture of exhilaration and absolute anxiety. It turned out to be an amazing night and it marked the start of our adult relationship.

However, it wasn't until I was in my mid-fifties that I finally found out why I have no memory of him living with my mum, my sister and me. He started the conversation by saying, 'Darling, I've got to tell you something …' I braced myself. Here was the truth. Before I was conceived, he had already left my mum and my sister for the woman who became his second wife and mother to my half-brother, the brilliant actor Jasper Britton. My father was handsome and couldn't resist women – and women found him equally irresistible, so there were lots of shenanigans even when he was with my mum. It transpired that during one visit of a few hours back to see her, he and my mum had temporarily rekindled their feelings and I was conceived. Did he go back to his new partner with a – possibly – guilty spring in his step? How did he manage to explain my eventual appearance to his future wife? And how did my mum tell her mum and brothers? I have no idea, but at least I had the truth. It fitted a huge piece of the jigsaw. He needed to get it off his chest and ultimately, I was grateful he did.

Looking back at these things, I can now see how easy it was to remove any sense of power from the little girl I was, without me even knowing it. And at the age of 55 I was left with a strong feeling of 'why did nobody say?' Everyone knew. My uncle, aunt, sister. They all knew. It was only me that was kept in the dark. As a result, I hate it when someone doesn't tell me what's going on. It upsets me and makes me very uneasy. I treasure people's honesty and frankness. I like to know where I am. These days, I will not be fobbed off when I try to find out what's going on. I yearn for the truth, even the worst kind of truth, as long as it is the truth. I also try hard to be sincere with people in return.

Trust is inevitably weakened after a revelation like that and this is the moment to lean on old friends for support. I am very lucky to have found friends whom I wholeheartedly trust and love and we can share all our difficult truths, knowing that it's not going anywhere else.

Old friends are fantastic, but finding new friends is also great. It keeps you young, engaged and excited. When you connect with someone unexpectedly, you perk up a bit. It creates a different rhythm to your routine. You don't know anything about each other, so there's a lot of 'tell me about yourself and I'll tell you a little about me'. You have no history, you're building it together, and suddenly you can be you. It's freeing and can give you a whole new perspective on life. Moving 300 miles away to Cornwall full-time created a huge physical distance between me and many good friends (thank goodness for Zoom and WhatsApp) but Cornwall is a friendly place and I was soon accepted into a new community. Only the other day my youngest daughter, Winnie, said: 'Mum, well done on making friends, being busy and not being a worry.' I'll take that as a win.

I would struggle way more if it weren't for my two great new friends, Boo and Two Cups. They are two of the most wonderful human beings. Funny, talented, kind. However tricky life seems, we are always there to bolster each other's self-belief. And I have learned that you can find new friends in the most unexpected places.

Boo and I arrived in our little village at the same time. Our houses have only one property in between us. I can stand and talk to her over the hedges. It was dogs that brought us together. She had a new puppy called Bailey and we had a three-year-old black Labrador called Denver.

While Bailey had heart-melting puppy eyes, Denver was handsome and well trained. He was not allowed on the sofa, not allowed upstairs and not allowed any titbits … until Phil was out of the house, at which point the girls and I would give him endless cuddles and the occasional digestive biscuit. Every evening I listened to *The Archers* on the sofa and if his master was not home yet, he'd hear the music and lie on top of me, with all four paws pointing skywards, while I tickled his tummy. The moment the closing music started, he'd jump off and go to his basket.

At that year's village fête there happened to be a dog show so Boo entered Bailey for Best Pup and I was confident that Denver would do very well in Most Handsome Dog. Blinking Bailey won his rosette but Denver came nowhere. Furious! But Boo and I have been friends ever since.

On another occasion, I was lured into taking part in our village flower and produce show. You wouldn't imagine a small community to have so many devoted and uber competitive exhibitors. My first entry was for my apples. Amazingly, they won first prize. Beginner's luck or was it the fact that I was the only entry in that class? It was during the show prizegiving that I became aware of a tall, slender blonde who looked like a rock chick and was being awarded 'first class' in almost every category. Her potatoes in a bucket, they won. Her miniature garden, that won. Her single rose was judged the best in show. Her flower arrangement: well, of course that triumphed too. Then she won two large cups AND the blooming first prize in the raffle as well. (All you need for a roast dinner.) It rather took the shine off my first-class apples. My friends Wyn and Toby had come down for the weekend and consoled me. 'Bloody "Two Cups"! Who does she think she is?' The name stuck.

(Now I think of it, there's a theme here. If you want to be my friend, you need to beat me in some kind of obscure competition.)

What can I tell you about my new pals? Well, Two Cups loves a vodka. It's her cure-all. She is also an incredible artist. She's a copyist, which is an artist who can copy a priceless original so brilliantly that no one would ever know. Her clients are never revealed but they are happy to put the real one in the bank while having a cracking fake above the baby grand. No one can tell the difference, even down to the signature. She's very knowledgeable and smart.

She also teaches at workshops, which Boo and I enjoy. How to paint like Matisse. Make shell hearts to hang on the wall. That sort of thing. And at Christmas she often does a wreath-making afternoon. There's music, wine, homemade shortbread and plenty of laughter. There was one class we joined which was about fish rubbing – I know, it does sound odd but really, it's fascinating. It's like printing but with a fish. It's inspired by the traditional Japanese art of *gyotaku*, dating from the 1800s, when fishermen took rubbings as a record of the fish they'd caught before their boat had docked, to illustrate their catch for customers. To do it, you put paint on the dead fish and then rub it with a cloth, before pressing down a sheet of rice paper on it and peeling back a beautiful print. I was so enjoying painting the fish that I never got to stage two. I got completely carried away, daubing it in all these gorgeous colours, even though the object was to make a print, not to have the most creatively coloured fish. It became quite the distraction for the class and then everyone was saying, 'I want to do what Fern's doing', instead of following instructions. I don't think I'll ever be allowed to another of her classes! Boo is also very creative and delivered the right kind of fish print.

Boo is incredibly elegant. She's got masses of lovely, long soft hair and a beautiful face. She dresses immaculately; classy and elegant even on a wet dog walk. Boo is just the kindest, most calm, organised person. She should be a therapist because she's so wise and also hilariously funny. She's a shining treasure of a friend, a jewel in our threesome. Two Cups and I can be quite full on, sometimes a bit arty and a bit silly, but Boo will always bring us back down to earth. Together we share the stories of our lives and try to offer solutions if asked for. The other day I sent a WhatsApp message telling them I was an idiot and the reply came back: 'You are an idiot, albeit a dear one.'

Having been in the public eye, meeting new people has a couple of difficulties. The first is that everyone knows my name but they never tell me theirs and it gets to a point in the conversation where I feel I can't ask, and the second is that I have a sort of face blindness. My father had it too. I can chat away to someone very happily but the next day I wouldn't remember their face at all. It's very embarrassing for me because it looks like I am being very rude. May I take this opportunity to apologise to those who I have ignored unintentionally? It takes me two or three meetings before I get it. But with Boo and Two Cups it was pretty instant. We're all complex women who've been through a lot. Between us we have eight children, five husbands and we have navigated very similar lives without having known each other for most of them. We came to this wonderful sort of 'waters meet' point where we've just coincided and we're together, while not having to constantly be in each other's company. We don't have to ring each other every day. We have a WhatsApp group and they're so effortlessly funny, their comments make me laugh out loud. Crucially, we don't have to pretend to be anything we're not.

Who knew that you could make new friends at this advanced age? Friends who bring back that marvellous stupidity, hope and faith of our teenage years. Well, you can. How? Don't hide away. Don't allow shyness, fear of ridicule or rejection stop you. It really is all too easy to hide away from the world – especially if you're feeling low or believe you don't have too much to offer – so it's important to remember that everyone feels some version of this. Yet each of us is really looking for the same thing – connection and people who make us feel 'part of the gang'. It's worth taking the risk with new people by putting ourselves out there. The only person who can do this is you.

Great friendships are such a boost and in turn they give you self-belief. After all, if someone wise and witty wants to spend time with you and really cares about you, then you can't be nearly as bad as that nagging voice in your head sometimes insists that you are. I never expected to find new friends in my sixties. Not that I really thought about it, but you know sometimes when you meet people and you just click? Now I feel extremely blessed. And happily, this fortu-itous bonding helped to add to my sense of Repowering.

The point in your life to begin Repowering is precisely where you are now. Most of us are brilliant procrastinators. I know I am, particularly when I'm writing a book. In the morning I'll think, *I'm going to sit down and write all day today.* Moments later, my good intentions crumble to dust when my powers of concentration falter. I'll think, *I'll just tidy that cupboard, then I'll spin around with the vacuum,* or

I might just do a bit of weeding for half an hour. It's a cliché because it's true. Writers really do have the cleanest houses.

Too often we sabotage ourselves by finding anything to do other than the thing we really want to be doing. I remember interviewing a wonderful American woman on *This Morning*. She was fantastic, full of great wisdom and knowledge. Nowadays she'd be doing a Ted Talk. Anyway, the thing that resonated most with me from our chat was when she said: 'The moment you say *but* is the moment you create drama in your life.' Isn't that good? If you hear yourself saying, 'Oh I'd love to *but* ...' you are stopping yourself with that little word. With three letters you've just created drama.

Procrastination happens for lots of reasons but for many of us it's that age-old dilemma of making perfection the enemy of good. Too many times we believe we can't do anything unless we accomplish it perfectly. We get involved with all sorts of negative self-talk and convince ourselves we aren't good enough to do whatever it is that needs to be done. We try so hard to get everything so brilliantly right that we end up tripping ourselves up and feeling exhausted and dejected.

Pop idol Donny Osmond has a great story about this. He is a consummate professional who has worked incredibly hard since he made his singing debut, aged five. He spent long days relentlessly rehearsing with his family. As an adult, he followed the same demanding schedule he learned in childhood, and he has always given his all. I saw that first-hand when we presented *This Morning* together once. He was fantastically slick. He was a great interviewer, in and out of breaks to the second. He was used to delivering perfection. But, he explained, it hadn't always been that easy, and it was an intervention by his wife Debbie that provided the answers.

A few years ago, when he was on tour, he was in the dressing room and suddenly had a complete meltdown. I guess it was some sort of panic attack. Everything just blew up for him. Debbie came in and found him very distressed. She held him and said, 'You know what you've got to do, Donny? You've got to go out there and just be average. Stop trying to be absolutely everything. Just be average and they won't even notice because your average is superb.' And it was.

After we did another show together, called *Fern Britton Meets …*, we had our photograph taken. Looking at it, I said mischievously, 'One of us needs plastic surgery.' Without missing a beat, he said, 'Well, it's not me.' I adore him. He's an example to us all.

Life has its ups and it has its downs, and there's no magic wand to make it all run along smoothly. There's also no way we can predict what's coming next. Just take comfort in the thought that we have muddled along this far and it's been

OK. Most of us are quite happy to dwell on all the things we've done badly or anywhere we've failed, whereas we rarely sit down and contemplate all the things we've done brilliantly. All the areas where we've excelled. You don't get to this sort of age without having a whole host of things that have worked out just fine.

I'm telling myself this as much as I'm saying it to you. It's a lesson I absolutely need to learn. I try so hard to practise self-compassion, but it doesn't come easily. If I see a bad review or something horrible written about me, all the good things I've achieved are as nothing and I start to beat myself up. I convince myself I am shite at everything. Why is it we only ever remember the negative stuff?

Here's a fine example. As a woman on television your entire being is discussed. Once, a male columnist – let's not be coy, his name is Tony Parsons – wrote that I looked 'like Moby Dick in a blonde wig ... Who really wants to see this obese old slapper wagging her enormous breasts at the camera?' Tony! I hope no one, man or woman, writes similarly about your own daughter.

The world can be ugly and people can be cruel, but that doesn't mean we have to be awful to ourselves. I'm sure you have examples of this in your life, too. Everyone's lovely at a party but perhaps someone says something a bit off and that's what stays with you. We really can be our own worst enemies. That awful internal voice can vocalise things to ourselves that we wouldn't in a million years say to a friend or even an acquaintance. That's why I work at trying to be nicer to myself. When it comes to self-compassion, I'm hoping practice makes perfect.

In learning to be kinder to myself, there are definite advantages. I've stopped feeling any guilt if I decide to make an appointment to have a manicure, pedicure, facial or to get my hair done. Those things take time out of a busy day and I used to feel so torn. Now, I tell myself I am quite within my rights to go and do it. I feel strongly that we have a duty to take care of ourselves and to give ourselves little treats. It doesn't have to be anything enormous; even a pasty on the beach on a nice day is enough to lift my spirits.

While belief in myself remains a work in progress, I have always had a faith in God but hadn't been a churchgoer for many years. Almost a year ago I decided to attend a Sunday service and see what our local church was like. I was met by the kindest, warmest and most welcoming group of people. I don't know what I was expecting but it was not what I found. It wasn't at all evangelical – there was no fire or brimstone – but I found it very engaging, with lots of great hymns, thoughtful prayer and laughs. Yes, laughs! In church! Who knew?

I am a Christian but not a very good example of one. I find going to church enormously settling. It's not a huge congregation, but the people are brilliant. They're funny, they're normal and no one is shoving questionable messages down anybody's throats. We're allowed to gently explore our faith and consequently, for me, that faith has developed. It had always been within me, but it's become easier to acknowledge now. When I returned after my three weeks in the *Celebrity Big Brother* house, slightly concerned that they had heard me swearing and behaving badly, one fellow churchgoer, a lovely man, put his arms around me and simply said, 'Welcome home.' Enough said.

Obviously I don't have all the answers. But I do recognise that all of us share a lot in common as we chart our course through life.

And so far, mine has been as confusing, complicated and discombobulating as everyone else's. It has been a series of amazing ups and excruciating downs, for sure. I had difficult years with a stepfather who always made me feel that little bit less than any child should feel. Then I left home and found my freedom before embarking on a sometimes exciting, sometimes awful TV career. I had lovely colleagues, and I had difficult ones. I went through gruelling IVF to have my amazing twin boys, went on to have my first daughter naturally, then I got divorced, I got remarried, and I had my last child at 44. And I imagine your life has been full of just as many positives and pitfalls.

But take a moment to look back and you can see that we navigated it all, with some measure of success. We emerged from our childhoods, braved our teens, stumbled through our responsible adult years, and perhaps marriages and parenthood. And now where are we? I'll tell you where we are. We're on the brink of a new and very different future. But we cannot do it unless we have faith and trust in ourselves.

Spread a Little Joy

Sometimes an apt quotation can provide a bit of inspiration for how to live your life. Here are some of my favourites:

- Captain John Ridgway – who rowed the Atlantic with Chay Blyth in 1966 – wrote in his book that we should 'always leave people and things better than you found them'.
- 'It's the courage to continue that counts.' That one is attributed to Winston Churchill.
- 'Love is patient and kind.' 1 Corinthians 13:4
- 'Do to others as you would have them do to you.' Luke 6:31

Chapter Three

We All Make Mistakes ...

*F*irst things first: we all make mistakes. A life without mess would not be worth living. The messy stuff in our lives challenges and teaches us. Failure is just a rehearsal for success.

When I think about making mistakes, Queen Camilla comes to mind. She's made a hell of a mess. So has the King. So has everybody. But she deserves praise now. Suddenly the King is ill and – bang! – she's right there, front and centre as if she were born to it. She owns the role and has such warmth and approachability. I guess that comes from not having lived a life that was all unimpeachable perfection. If, like me, you're looking beyond your sixties into your seventies, then she's an icon. She and I share a birthday, but Camilla's ten years older than me. She's taken on the biggest job of her life in her seventies. It is almost as if she is the poster girl for Repowering.

But Camilla is proof that no one will have got through life without having made mistakes. There's that awful expression – *failure isn't an option*. Well actually, it's not only an option but an inevitability. Whether it's reversing into a bollard, inadvertently spilling the beans on something that's meant to be top secret, accidentally insulting someone, going on a disastrous date against your better judgement, marrying the wrong person or perhaps not paying attention to one of your children when they really need it. The list is endless. Life is chaotic and there's nothing any of us can do to change that. I've a strong feeling that your mind is wandering back to that last time you made an excruciating error. Mine, too. Let me share a couple of the worst examples with you now.

Once at work we did a programme live from an airport over an entire weekend. Afterwards, there was a huge group of us in a big room. We were talking over how it had gone and a man I hadn't met before said something like, 'Well, it was a ridiculous programme to have done anyway because ...'

I took umbrage at his flippant remark, so instantly I took him to task. Somewhat loftily, I said: 'Well, clearly you don't understand the aviation industry.'

He gave me a long, hard stare before replying: 'I run the RAF base in Belize.'

There I was, trying to be cocky, and I got squashed. Quite rightly. I had no choice but to apologise.

I'm lucky that I have had the kind of jobs where most of my mistakes generally cause only huge humiliation for me, and nothing more dire than that. Some days are better than others, and sometimes it seems like we can't do right for doing wrong. Here is one example of being a working mum with an eye off the ball.

It started when I came home from a long day on *This Morning*. I fed the children, bathed them, read stories and put them to bed. Phew, now it was my time to relax. But a little while later, when I expected them to be sound asleep, the boys – who were about nine at the time – wandered down. One of them looked at me earnestly and said: 'By the way, Mum, it's evacuee day at school tomorrow.' Then the other one chipped in: 'Yeah, we can't wear our uniforms; we have to go dressed as Second World War evacuees.'

By this point it was rapidly heading towards 9.30pm and I had to be up at 4.45am. And now I had to throw together two 1940s outfits *and* era-appropriate lunches. We scrambled around and eventually discovered a scrunched-up note from school in one of the boys' book bags. The instructions were specific. *Lunch boxes should preferably contain sandwiches made from homemade bread and should contain nothing that would have been unavailable during wartime. Clothing must be authentic for the period.*

Every mother, I'm sure, has experienced something like this, whether it's an unexpected bake sale or having to produce a working model of a volcano in the dying hours of the night.

As luck would have it, my mum was on hand to offer advice. Desperately looking around the kitchen for food I could put in their lunch box, I said: 'I can put a banana in, can't I?'

'No,' she said, quickly. 'We didn't have bananas during the war.'

Crisps? No, we didn't have crisps. Chocolate? No, we didn't have chocolate. I briefly considered grating a carrot before remembering the boys didn't like carrots.

Fortunately, their paternal grandmother was a very good knitter, so when it came to kitting the boys out we had lots of homemade jumpers which were perfect. I found some grey shorts that barely fitted them, but they just about worked. So at least, I thought, that was sorted. They'd have to make do with 21st-century shoes and socks but surely as I'd made the effort it would all be OK.

Helpful advice was coming thick and fast from my mother, like: 'They need a gas mask around their necks, and it should be in a brown cardboard box, tied with string.'

To my immense credit, I managed a smile before suggesting she head off home. The next morning, I got up early and Super Sue, our nanny, came in at 6am, just as I was about to get in the car to go to work. At this time, Winifred, who was still a baby, came to work with me because I was breast-feeding, so I'd already got her washed and changed, and was ready to leave.

As we passed the baton, I said to Super Sue: 'It's evacuee day at school today so I've set out their clothes.' (I'd laid them out on the floor in the bedroom in the shape of little humans.) 'Their lunches are in the fridge, wrapped in greaseproof paper.'

Feeling rather smug, I arrived at the *This Morning* studio and learned we were doing an item on vibrators. This was fine, except we weren't allowed to say 'vibrators' and we were absolutely not allowed to say 'dildos' under any circumstances. We were permitted to say 'sex toys' or something similarly anodyne.

So, there we were, live on television, trying very, very hard not to say those two words. Except that the expert I was interviewing kept saying the 'd'-word and I had to repeatedly say, 'So, sorry, can we call them sex toys?' To which she would reply, 'Yes, yes, of course – so this dildo is ...'

Anyway, we got through it and I thought, *Phew! Could have been worse.* Next up, though, was an interview with a beautiful model-turned-actress who was on tour with *The Vagina Monologues.* (There was definitely an overarching theme going on that day!) Well, we were chatting away, and then she said: 'There are lots of actresses in the play. We each do a small part. I have my own monologue ...'

There was a pause ...

'It's called "Reclaiming Cunt".'

I can still feel the flush of panic and the urge to laugh rise through me as the words left her mouth and I tried to keep my cool as the interview continued. Among friends, I am an excellent swearer, but never would I ever swear on daytime television. The next day in a newspaper someone wrote that the 'presenters appeared not to notice'. I guess that's a lesson in itself. We might think we've made an awful mess of something, but the rest of the world is often oblivious.

Anyway, the day from hell didn't stop there. I'd survived the dildos and the C-word but, at the end of the show, while the team was having the usual debrief and finding it all hilarious, I suddenly remembered I had to present a prize to the Nurse of the Year at the *Daily Mail* NHS Heroes awards ceremony. Unfortunately, I couldn't remember where it was taking place. I couldn't remember what time. I couldn't remember anything at all.

So, I scooped up Winifred, rushed outside and jumped into the car and, after a couple of frantic phone calls, my driver Tony managed to get us to the venue in Kensington. As soon as we pulled up at the kerb, I jumped out clutching Winnie, already 20 minutes late. Panting, I arrived at the reception desk only to be told the awards ceremony was up a flight of stairs, down a long corridor, through some doors …

I ran all the way and, as I flung open the double doors, a man on the stage at the other end of the room said, 'And here she is now …'

I threw Winifred at Lynn Faulds Wood, the consumer journalist, who was another guest at the event. I knew her a little because her husband, John Stapleton, had worked with my first husband, Clive, on TV-am and I had met her on *Breakfast Time* way back in the 1980s. I hadn't seen her for years but, when I ran into the room, flustered and out of breath, she said, 'Give me the baby.' I ran to the stage and made it up there in a flurry of forced smiles and extravagant apologies.

Standing there, in front of a room full of expectant faces, all I could think was, *I don't know the name of the award or the name of the person I'm presenting it to.* So I stepped away from the mic and went across to the man at the end of the stage. 'I'm so sorry,' I whispered, 'but I can't remember what the prize is and who it's going to.'

I was perspiring profusely and by now I wasn't even sure how to walk any more, such was the effect of raging panic. As always, I continued to plaster on a smile. I smile a lot; I have had a smiley face since I was little. I remember the girl next door, when we were about five or six, asking, 'Why do you smile all the time?' It's the dolphins' curse. Dolphins always look like they are smiling, whereas inside they might be really miserable. There's a Cat Stevens song, 'Wild World', which claims it's hard to get by just upon a smile. Well, no, it's not actually. You can do it.

Anyway, the man at the side of the stage handed me a piece of paper and I went back to the microphone – and it was at that moment I realised I hadn't got my reading glasses. I had to shuffle back across the stage for a second time and ask the man to read it aloud to me. By now I was ludicrously over-compensating, telling the patient nurse that had come up onto the stage that she was the most perfect person I had ever met. I started hyperventilating when I noticed the journalist Lynda Lee-Potter in the audience, one of the *Daily Mail's* columnists. *Oh God*, I thought. *Maybe she'll write about this horrible catastrophe in tomorrow's paper.*

She had once written a piece commenting on my sepa-ration from my first husband along the lines that I should stay married and cosy in my size 16 dresses. Princess Diana described her as 'one of the Wednesday witches' (as most female newspaper columns were published on a Wednesday). In fact, Lynda was a fine person, but everyone in the glare of the media spotlight remembers the worst reviews they've ever had, and many of them were penned by her.

As I got off the stage – shaking and sweating, and thinking, *I just want to go home* – a waiter said, 'I'll show you to your seat,' which was, of course, next to Lynda Lee-Potter. She was the last person I wanted to make small talk with when I was feeling like the most incompetent person in the world. However, she was sweet to me. Thank heaven for small mercies!

Lynn Faulds Wood handed Winnie back to me and I made my excuses and left. Hugely apologetic after my series of howlers, I said, 'I'm so sorry, but I have to get the baby home.'

Was this the end to a sorry day? Oh no. In the car I had a blissful few moments congratulating myself on getting away with it. *Aargh, it's finally all over. What an effing awful day.* Then my maternal instincts kicked in and I thought I'd ring home to make sure everything was OK.

Super Sue answered the phone. 'Oh, hi Fern,' she said. 'You do know it wasn't evacuee day today, don't you?'

'What?'

'It's tomorrow. I felt such a fool taking them to school dressed like that when everyone else was in uniform.'

Every single working mother in the world has had a day like this.

This story also reminds me of when I had my own wardrobe malfunction as a schoolgirl. One Tuesday morning we were running late for swimming and my mum suggested I put my swimming costume on under my uniform so I could make it into the pool on time. I did just that and enjoyed my swimming lesson immensely. But in the changing room afterwards, I rummaged through my bag and I realised I had no underwear.

My school skirt was relatively short and pleated, but I thought I'd get away with not wearing any knickers until home time. (It wasn't like I had any other options.) Later that breezy day we went out to the quad, as usual. For some reason I was jumping from bench to bench and, of course, my skirt went up like a parachute and everyone could see I didn't have any underwear on. It was mortifying and I can honestly say I have never again forgotten my knickers. Fortunately when it came to the knickers, it was an all girls' school.

Being knickerless is not the only memory that makes me cringe with mortification. Again, when I was a teenager, one member of the family lived in a village where there was a school for the blind. It was a boarding school and, because parents couldn't get to visit their children every weekend, families in the village would befriend children and have them over for tea or take them out.

My relation befriended this lovely girl called Maureen and it was decided we should meet her too. So, me, my mum and my stepfather went over to have afternoon tea. The conversation was a little stilted as we'd only just met, but biscuits and sandwiches were being handed round and we were all working hard to keep the conversation going. I have no idea how it happened, but when the plate of biscuits got to me, I passed it to Maureen and – with the words getting horribly jumbled in my mouth – I said, 'Biscuit, moron?'

It was so utterly appalling, the worst thing. I have no idea how it even came out of my mouth. I went bright red and began to sweat. Maureen didn't appear to have noticed. She just took a biscuit and the afternoon continued. I ummed and ahhed about telling you this because it's too awful but I also wanted to reassure you that we all do inexplicable things every now and then. I don't know about you, but when I make a mistake of that magnitude I feel sort of prickly on the inside and I want to disappear. Even now, it makes me cringe to think about it and I feel sick to my stomach.

There are phases you go through after you make a mistake. It's a bit like grief, in a way. Disbelief – surely I didn't just do that? Anger – how could I have been so stupid? Denial – perhaps no one noticed. Bargaining – if time could miraculously be turned back, I promise to be perfect for the rest of my life. And finally, acceptance – yup, I am capable of doing some quite outrageously stupid things. But hey, I'm also capable of doing some great things too, so it all balances out in the end.

As I've grown older, I've consoled myself with the knowledge that making mistakes is an intrinsic part of being human. Some of them are tiny, some of them huge. Some of them funny, some mortifying. We do it from the moment we start to walk and talk. Whatever they are and however old we are when we make them, they are learning opportunities. It's our failures as much as our successes that shape our identities and make us who we are. They also help us to become more resilient and teach us how to succeed.

No matter how deeply ashamed you feel, after a while you generally have to laugh. That's just what happens when you are British. There is something funny in most mistakes and the ability to laugh at ourselves is one of our greatest achievements. It takes practice but, honestly, once you can do it, life is so much easier.

The aviation man I can laugh about and the day from hell is now a great dinner party story. I will never, ever get over Maureen and the biscuits, though.

For centuries, society has been quick to shame women for EVERYTHING. We really have got to stop it. We are what we are. I have decided not to feel ashamed about who I am or how I look. Shame is a heavy weight to carry through a life. Put it down. See yourself as you really are. A human passing through. Wanting all the things everybody wants. Love. Security. A roof over your head. Food in your tummy and enough money to keep you going. I appreciate everybody's 'enough' is different. For some it would be to have a million pounds in the bank, for others just a home to go back to.

Separating our mistakes from ourselves is essential because when we don't do this it has real potential to damage our self-worth and self-esteem. When we internalise mistakes, we start to see them as part of us and they intertwine with our identity. It's no longer an isolated incident but it becomes, in our heads, a reflection of our inherent flaws and incompetence.

It doesn't end there. We will inevitably start to use language to ourselves that no one wants to hear, like 'clumsy', 'stupid' and 'ridiculous', and it's enough to trigger a downward spiral. Here's a quick hack to help. Instead of saying, 'I'm an idiot' or 'I'm such a failure', be more dispassionate and disconnect behaviour from judgement. Rather than saying, 'I failed', say, 'That attempt failed.' Don't declare, either to yourself or the world, that you are a fool; instead say, 'Well, that was a foolish thing I did.' Do you see the difference? Reframing our perspective like this allows us to be objective about ourselves and the mistakes we make. It also allows us to feel compassion for ourselves, which is important when we're feeling awful about something that has just happened.

Some mistakes are emotional, some are financially ruinous and some are simply physical. In March 2020 – just as lockdown happened – I was taking a big black bag of rubbish to the wheelie bin. As I approached the bin, a random thought popped into my head: *Ooh, I used to be quite good at shot put at school.* Only one thing filled my mind now: could I replicate the skill and finesse I'd had in the old days on the school playing fields? And that's why I attempted to throw the bag – which was hanging down my back like Father Christmas's sack – into the bin as if I were doing shot put.

Unfortunately, at no point immediately prior to the big throw were illusions about my sporting prowess dislodged by memories of my poor grasp of physics. I opened the bin lid and thrust the bag forward. But instead of a sense of childish achievement I felt an immediate searing pain. Instantly,

I knew I'd done something serious. For over a year I was in agony and it was at the time when you really couldn't see a doctor. Eventually I got to see a fantastic NHS surgeon who told me I had to have a total shoulder replacement. I was so relieved that he knew I wasn't making the pain up, I cried. I had to wait a year for the op but it was so worth it. It gave me time to get fit again, but more of that later.

To my children, I have laid bare my worst mistakes as I think it's important to highlight that they are a natural part of life. Winifred has embraced the idea of mistakes so whole-heartedly that she's gathering my stories, her own and her sister's, and compiling them all into a book. One day, I hope you'll read it.

I really like Winnie's approach. It seems to me to be incredibly healthy. You must make a choice in life: decide to embrace your mistakes or get crushed by them. If we can do the former, I think we get over them much more quickly. Tell the stories of your shame and watch them turn into hilarious family anecdotes. The people who are important love us regardless of the mistakes we make.

However, sometimes in life we make truly terrible mistakes that we can't laugh off and that hurt people very badly. We might call them 'home truths' which we deliver with the best possible intentions, but they inevitably leave wreckage on the emotional highway. Over the years I have, like everyone else, unthinkingly hurt people. I've also spoken to others who have crushed the hearts of those they love and it has inevitably been incredibly difficult to rebuild those relationships, and also to forgive themselves.

All I can repeat here is the adage that you can't do better until you know better. You must try very hard to forgive yourself, and others, and it won't be easy. Trying to understand why you did what you did is a good place to start and if you're feeling so wretched it's interfering with all aspects of your life, it might be useful to talk to a professional.

Time does heal and, in most situations, it is rarely a clear case of anyone being an outright villain. Life is more nuanced than that. Whatever you may have done or feel you're responsible for, it really shouldn't hold you back from being your best self again. If you allow yourself to be swallowed up by guilt and regret, you'll hurt not only yourself but those close to you, too.

It's also important to keep some perspective. You didn't accidentally shoot down a jumbo jet – hopefully not, anyway. Nobody died. Forgive yourself and others will forgive you. This sounds trite but it's true. Of course, be sorry if you've done something awful and, of course, do everything you can to put things right if you've hurt or upset someone, but don't go on about it forever. It helps no one. On the odd occasion your attempt to make amends is not deemed good enough by the other person, then you must move on. I know it might sound cruel but you've tried your hardest, it hasn't worked, so for the sake of all concerned it's best just to walk away.

If you can forgive yourself, offer that same generosity of spirit to others. People will do things that are hurtful. They'll be careless with our possessions and our hearts at times. It doesn't mean they're a terrible person. It simply is what it is. At times we cannot help ourselves and neither can others. All we can do is our best and that's all we can hope for from them, too.

Give people the benefit of the doubt. When someone is snappy or short, remember that we don't know exactly what's going on with them. They might be unwell. They might be suffering something awful at home. They might just be plain exhausted. It's rarely you at the centre of their personal tempest. Something unconnected that's happening for them is at the root of their issues. When I've been unkind to somebody at work (rarely, I hope), I have always made a point of apologising afterwards. On the odd occasion it's happened, it's been in the heat of the moment. The good thing about getting older is that temperamental flare-ups aren't so easily provoked.

There are two kinds of worry attached to mistakes. The anxiety about something we've already done and the worry of something pending, like making a tricky choice. This kind of stress induces high anxiety. It's the sort of thing that keeps us up at night. Understandably so, as big decisions are a tough call. We worry about plumping for the wrong option and can get ourselves into a stultifying state of fretfulness.

I once made a horrible error in taking the wrong job. I'd been working for a theatre company as a stage manager and I loved it. I quickly rose from assistant stage manager to deputy stage manager. I worked very closely with the director Jonathan Lynn and all the actors, which I loved. Jonathan always had abundant talent. He's worked in London's theatreland, on Broadway, in television and has made feature films. Still, he would ask for my opinion on the actors' performances. He would listen to my answers and that boosted my confidence. I found myself thinking I'd quite like to be a director myself, and daydreamed that maybe this was a role he had in mind for me.

Then, out of the blue, he called me into his office and offered me the position of marketing officer for the company. He told me he thought I'd be good at it. So I took the job. Even before I said 'yes', I was worried about it as I wouldn't be working with actors any more, which was a part of my working life I loved. Instead, I would go ahead of the company to the next place a performance was scheduled and it would be my job to drum up business.

I was flattered into taking the job, but it was such a mistake. I was lonely. I missed the actors and being in the theatre. In fact, I missed everything about my old job and liked nothing about the new one. I stayed for a while, but then I couldn't take it any more.

I quit and was out of work for four weeks. All that time, my stepfather kept telling me I couldn't 'go on the dole'. I didn't. I went on to get my first job in television So it all worked out in the end.

On the one hand, a bad decision – a mistake – led me on to a career I loved. On the other hand, if I had stayed, perhaps I would be a director by now. I might have an amazing play on at the National! I'm laughing as I type this, because I don't for a minute believe that could be true, but you know what I mean. Essentially, what I'm saying is that if we make the wrong decision, the chances are it will work out anyway. Maybe not in the way we had initially thought but it might just take us down another path.

Mistakes can be inspirational. Some of the greatest inventions ever have come out of what would have initially been seen as a mistake. The Post-it note was only launched in 1980 because someone trying to invent a strong adhesive managed instead to produce a weak but peelable one. Play-Doh was meant to be a wallpaper cleaner for homes with sooty domestic fires. When coal went out of favour, the compound was repackaged for children. Even the humble Slinky had a previous life, keeping sensitive ship equipment steady in turbulent waters. It never found its sea legs but what child hasn't spent a joyous afternoon watching one shimmy down the stairs?

Being open to making mistakes makes us more robust. In the face of failure, we are presented with a choice: to succumb to despair or to rise above adversity. Those who embrace their mistakes as part of the journey understand that setbacks are not permanent, but rather temporary obstacles that can be overcome with determination and perseverance. The result is renewed resilience, and each mistake we make strengthens our ability to bounce back even stronger than before.

When we allow ourselves the freedom to make mistakes, we open the door to new possibilities. By embracing a mindset of experimentation and exploration, we can uncover unexpected solutions. It's also worth remembering that mistakes can foster humility and empathy. When we're reminded of our own fallibility and imperfection it often encourages us to be a little bit more compassionate and understanding of others. Through these, sometimes appalling, situations, our relationships are often deepened.

Sometimes just the fear of making a mistake can be paralysing and can hamper us from making big decisions. If you're on the cusp of a significant decision, it is a good idea to think about how it might affect your life in three months, six months, a year, five years. Will it still matter then? You can't Repower your life without making some changes and you can't make changes without making decisions. Even if that decision is to change nothing big right now. Bear in mind, too, that small, incremental changes can be as power-ful as a momentous life-changing one.

For example, you might want fitness to play a big part in your new life, but don't feel ready or able to join a gym. There's no reason, though, not to add some walking into your life. Whether it's factoring in a walk each evening or just getting off the bus a stop or so earlier on your way to work, it can make a big difference in boosting your fitness levels and confidence. Gold medallist Keely Hodgkinson describes athletic achievement as being 10 per cent physical and 90 per cent mental. Just let that sink in for a moment.

If something is genuinely too big for you, your heart will tell you you're not ready. The trick is working out whether it's your heart or your fear talking. If you think it'll be very challenging, but you'd like to try, then go for it. Have confi-dence in yourself. Failure is only a rehearsal for success. I can be quite impulsive when it comes to big decisions and have regretted that at times, so lately I have tried to slow myself down, to take a beat, to sleep on it, to quietly think about it before rushing in.

Some things are too big to decide on your own and asking for help is perfectly fine. In fact, it's a good idea. After all, if you know your house needs rewiring but are not an electrician, the only way it's going to get done safely is to call in a professional. It's the same with most big things in life. If your relationship feels as if it's over or you want to make a life-changing career decision, then there's absolutely no shame in seeing a counsellor to talk it over. In fact, it makes an awful lot of sense to get in a professional who has no vested interest in your life to help you work through the pros and cons of any big decision.

And if that decision goes a bit wrong, that's OK too. When we make a mistake or fail at something, we have a choice. We can either shuffle away and hide, abandoning all hope of success, or face up to the issue, be honest with those around us and regroup to think of our next steps before eventually trying again. It's like that with any element of Repowering. If we decide to get fit but just can't face a run in the rain, or if we resolve to fix our diet but are seduced by a huge bar of chocolate, it doesn't matter as long as we don't see it as a reason to give up the overall goal. This all-or-nothing thinking is often what keeps us in a loop of failure.

Instead, if we own our mistakes and see them as steps on a journey, making a point of reassuring ourselves that any setbacks we encounter are not permanent, then we're way more likely to achieve whatever it is we're hoping for. What can we learn from our error? Perhaps it's to make sure we don't have any chocolate in the cupboard, or maybe to check the weather before we make an exercise plan for the week. Although I actively enjoy running, swimming or cycling in the rain!

It's also good to acknowledge that most of us have no idea at all what we're doing. We're just winging it and trying to get by. If we're lucky enough to have good friends, then they will provide a safe landing if we fall. When I look at Boo and Two Cups, I think they are amazing. They're holding their lives together, with adult children, partners, work and a busy lifestyle. And behind all this great stuff, I know they're just like me and are thinking, *I don't know what the f**k I'm doing! I don't have a clue at all.*

It's very easy to be hobbled by shame, by fear … by, you know, that desperate, clawing feeling of 'please don't recognise that I did that'. Then you cut off your friends who would probably love to make you feel much better about whatever it was that went wrong. It's much healthier just to 'fess up to it and say, 'Yes, I mucked up.' It makes you feel better, but it also makes the people around you feel better too, perhaps because they're thrilled it didn't happen to them or because they get to say, 'Well done, you – now let's move on.' So don't drag suitcases full of bad choices around with you. They'll weigh you down. I've only now – in my sixties – started to leave old mistakes behind and it really is fabulously liberating …

Find Your Way with Fern

- My mum always said that what you have on your feet shows on your face. Comfort over pain every time!

- She also said that it's never your extravagances you regret, it's your economies (this is the best excuse for buying something that blows the budget).

- When my children were small I could forgive their mistakes the first time because 'you don't know until you know'. But if they made the same mistake again they'd be in trouble.

- I think it's probably best to only ever admit to five previous boyfriends or lovers.

- And finally, never, never get drunk on cheap champagne – the next day is death. See the second point above!

Chapter Four

Imposter Syndrome

*E*ver felt like a phony? I've always thought that people who know what they are doing can look right through me and know I'm nothing more than a great pretender. That's never been truer for me than with writing.

I've written 11 novels, an autobiography and several cookery books, and I'm a *Sunday Times* number one best-selling author. All that is true but I find it hard to say it out loud. If there was a literary emergency and someone yelled, 'Is there a writer in the house?', I wouldn't put my hand up. I have only just put that as my occupation on a new passport and when I went through passport control in America, the man gave me a hard stare before saying, 'You're an author?' I was about to confess shamefacedly, 'No, I'm not really.' Then he smiled and said, 'That must be very interesting.'

This is a real example of imposter syndrome. The persistent whisper in the back of our minds, undermining any achievements we've notched up and casting doubt on our abilities. It can be triggered by taking on a new job. And I am 100 per cent sure it is particularly unrelenting among writers.

I contrast myself with 'proper' authors, like Kate Atkinson, for instance. For me, she is an expert in the art. She thinks of different plots and distinctive characters while I very much rely on Cornwall and the stuff I know. At the start of my writing career, this was a saving grace for me. I was in a place I loved. The landscape was nourishing, and it helped me focus on moving forward. And still, Cornwall is for me the perfect place to be. My novels find their roots in the gentle rhythm of life down here and it feels like home territory. But should I look for more?

'The worst enemy to creativity is self-doubt,' said writer Sylvia Plath, and I agree. When you have produced a book, everyone cautions you against looking at the reviews. But, always against my better judgement, I can't help but check out the reader reviews from time to time. Lovely words like 'wit', 'warmth' and 'wisdom' I cannot take on board, but one review I got for my 2022 book, *The Good Servant*, began with the words: 'In the end, I decided that this is quite a good book.' OK, I could take that. It concluded by saying, 'The tale is a compelling and affecting one, that might have been better in the hands of a more accomplished writer.' I took that, too. This was a person who knew I was sh*t and said it. Why do I feel more comfortable with that lukewarm review? Is it something to do with being British? I can't take too much ego boosting. I'd much prefer to be told, 'You're OK,' than, 'Oh, you shine, you're the best, this is incredible.' No, my brain has an allergy to that; I just can't accept it.

The Good Servant was something of a departure for me, writing about a real woman, Marion Crawford, rather than fictional ones. She was the governess to Queen Elizabeth II and Princess Margaret and was better known to them as Crawfie. She delayed her own marriage for 16 years so as not to abandon King George VI and his family, and only left service after the wedding of Elizabeth and Prince Philip. When she wrote a generous book about the young Royals, she was ostracised by them and died alone and heartbroken.

Maybe when I was younger, I would have given up all thoughts of attempting to write another book after that review, but with age comes resilience and I got over it. However, it has taken me a couple of years to deliver the next novel. When I am having those feelings of self-doubt, I can always talk to Boo or Two Cups, who have been friends with me long enough to know that they can laugh at me. Boo will always pour me a Cosmo and for Two Cups, it will always be a vodka.

At its core, imposter syndrome stems from a distorted perception of our accomplishments and abilities. When we experience imposter syndrome we often dismiss our achievements as luck or timing rather than acknowledging the skills we have and the hard work we've put in – despite external validation and tangible evidence that we're a success. It is awful and can lead us to avoid new challenges or opportunities due to fear of failure or being exposed as 'a fraud'.

Even Meryl Streep, a fellow sufferer, was once quoted as saying, 'Why would anyone want to see me again in a movie? And I don't know how to act anyway, so why am I doing this?' Jennifer Lopez once admitted: 'Even though I had sold 70 million albums, there I was feeling like I'm no good at this.'

When it was first identified in the 1970s, imposter syndrome was believed to be something that only affected successful women. Now it's known it can impact anyone and research points to 70 per cent of people experiencing it during their lives. Although it's not a diagnosable mental disorder it can lead to anxiety, which in itself may beckon in depression.

One striking aspect remains, which is how often it hits high achievers. Weirdly, the more successful someone becomes, the more intensely those feelings can kick in.

While many of us experience imposter syndrome, it's important not to let it stop us doing what we want to do. The world would be a much poorer place if we didn't get to watch Meryl Streep act in movies or sing along with J-Lo and the same would apply if you didn't get to do what you have your heart set on. Imposter syndrome is hard to cope with, yes, but feelings aren't facts. Just because we feel we're going to fail or aren't good enough, it doesn't mean it's true.

I was 52 when I left *This Morning* and it wasn't easy. I knew I had to go for lots of reasons, not least that I was getting on a bit. I wasn't too sure what would happen next, but as fate would have it I segued almost immediately into writing, which is now my bread and butter. It's been a huge learning process for me and although it hasn't been easy by any means, it's been worth it. Writing is incredibly hard work. I said to my son the other day I'd rather do 72 hours of non-stop live broadcasting than sit down and do 30 minutes in front of the computer, which on that day at that time was how I felt. However, when writing is going well, there is nothing like it; to see words coming from your own imagination and sticking to a page is mind-blowing. Sometimes when I close my laptop for the day and return the next morning to review yesterday's work, I can't remember writing what I see. It's like the shoemaker and the elves. The shoemaker goes to bed, leaving piles of unmade shoes, and comes down to find them finished, all by the elves he never sees.

I still get in a complete muddle with plotlines although that doesn't reduce me to tears any more. When you find your brain can't figure out the problem in front of you, the trick is to empty your mind, stop thinking about the problem at hand and find something completely different to do for that moment. Go and clear out a wardrobe or go for a walk. Anything that is not the problem. You'll be surprised at how your subconscious will be working by itself on the answer. Recently, someone asked me if I was still *churning out* novels. I could have clattered them. Churning implies it's easy, like turning a handle. It's far from that. I was lucky that it worked out, though. Sometimes a new job is not a matter of choice and that makes it all the more daunting, but possibly all the more rewarding.

Imposter syndrome, with its attendant plummet in confidence, can hit at any age, and parenting styles might play a part. When you're young, if you're not given approval and enthusiasm and aren't told 'you can do that', it can be very harmful. I'm not saying I was damaged by my parents, although it was sometimes a tricky upbringing. But as an example, when I published a cookbook, I showed it to my mum and she simply said, 'Oh, it's a book.' I said: 'What did you expect – a school project? A folder with A4 sheets I've drawn on and coloured in?' When I first told my father I'd got a job as a television continuity announcer, he said, 'Well, you're too fat to be Sue Lawley.' That kind of thing sticks with you.

I try to take heed of the experiences of others. I was listening to the radio the other day and a woman was asked if she ever felt nervous. She replied: 'If I am invited into the room, it's because I have a place in it.' That's smart and spot-on thinking.

You might very well ask why I decided to become a writer, given this underlying lack of conviction. Well, after my autobiography was published, another publishing company asked me to write a novel and I said, 'I don't think I can.' There's a huge difference between writing the script for a news item (as I used to do in my first job) and the contents of a 100,000-word novel, I told them. They said, 'No, honestly, give it a go.' Being brutally honest, the only reason I accepted the offer in the first place was because my children were approaching A-levels and university and I thought this would help me pay their university fees so they didn't have to come out with huge debt. But the publisher allocated to me an editor who firmly held my hand and got me through it. She was always there to pick me up and mop my tears. She'd send me chocolate and vodka. And she could, in a sentence, untangle the mess of the story in my head.

She gave me one piece of advice that I'm passing on to any aspiring writers out there. She told me: get over the first sentence, you are unlikely to emulate the famous first lines that have earned a place in literary history. You can't write, 'Last night I dreamt I went to Manderley again.' That was purloined just before the Second World War by Daphne du Maurier in her novel *Rebecca*. 'Happy families are all alike;

every unhappy family is unhappy in its own way.' Powerful stuff but already taken, by Leo Tolstoy for his novel *Anna Karenina*, sixty years before that. First lines are important but it's counterproductive to spend too much time pondering them, my editor revealed. She was brilliant as my editor and has moved on to be brilliant elsewhere.

On the second book, the people at the publishers said, 'Off you go!' It was like having stabilisers off a bike for the first time. Although I remained wobbly, I knew I could do it and, crucially, so did they. I now have a lovely new editor helping me with the next novel and another helping me with this book. The wonderful thing about editors is how absolutely invested they are in you and the writing and the characters and the plot and the birth of the book. They are with you all the way, like a midwife. But, as a midwife can't have a baby for you, an editor can't write the story, nor can they tell you how or where it's going to end.

But only this morning my fiction editor sent me an email, saying, *I am here to help and I'm undaunted by fixing things – that's my job.* It has really picked me up, the assurance that someone was on hand to help. It's the same in most jobs, but sometimes I think we feel a bit embarrassed asking. But when we do ask for assistance, it tends to make us feel better. Just getting over that slight fear of doing so takes some courage. The point is that when we start to Repower our careers or any other area of our life, it's rare that we're alone. Often we can find amazing, inspiring women to help us if we're willing to lean on them.

I usually write about relationship dynamics, like first romances, mid-life couplings and competitive relationships with siblings. Universal themes that are relevant to so many of us because they are daily facets of our lives. In examining them I can often relate them to my own life and that has certainly helped me move forward. Consciously or otherwise, writers use familiar ideas with which they can sympathise or empathise. One good example for me is a character missing a father. As I write, I wonder what it would have been like to sit on his shoulders or have a hug with him.

When I wrote *Daughters of Cornwall*, which became my best-selling book, a lot of the plotlines were easily at hand. It had transpired that my grandmother, a tough, strong, loving, kind woman, had given birth to a baby before she was married, and paid to have him privately fostered. I found out while I was working at Westward Television in 1981, when I received a letter from a man who said he was my uncle. I asked him for evidence before bringing this bombshell to my mother, and he provided a birth certificate, some letters in my grandmother's handwriting and photos that confirmed a family resemblance. When I told her, my mother wasn't unduly surprised. Years before, when my grandmother was dying, she had told her children she'd done something awful, a confession they took as confused ramblings. Now it seems like she was looking for an answer for feelings of guilt. She was a wonderful mother and grandmother. She was our nana. We used to watch Saturday-afternoon wrestling on the television together, while I would count the contents of her button box. When I was writing *Daughters of Cornwall*, I wanted to tell her story, to show that she did what she had to do; to find yourself pregnant and unmarried in the 1920s was not easy.

Hidden Treasures, written in 2012, is about someone who leaves London and throws herself into country life, finding a new set of eccentric friends. But although I might know something of the circumstances in this book and in other plotlines, I never base the characters on people I know. I just couldn't do it.

With writing, there's a process and for me it starts in my office, which overlooks the garden and isn't far from the log burner. For me it helps to work with my internal clock. I'm a morning person, so I'm always at my desk early. That way I can start writing when my brain is at its busy best. I work in complete silence. How I envy my artist pal, Two Cups, who can produce a wonderful work of art while listening to a podcast or an audiobook. I set myself a cut-off time in which I try to write 1,000 words, but sometimes the morning goes and I only have 200 words on the page in front of me. Then I'll give myself a break. This might, I admit, entail watching *Bargain Hunt* or *Homes Under the Hammer*.

People often ask me if live television is harder than writing and the answer is always a resounding no. It's absolutely the other way round. In a studio, you're part of a big team. There's always a buzz. People are always coming in and asking questions. Meetings can be anywhere. The make-up room, over lunch or on the phone. Now, suddenly, it is just me in my own little office with a laptop and a blank Word document blinking away.

People, I think, find writing exotic, more so somehow than television because it's all done behind closed doors. Everyone thinks they know how television works, even though it's nothing like it looks on the screen. Books are like a kind of alchemy because there's nothing and then there's this tangible something.

It's taken quite a while, but I've found a new rhythm. I'm much better at organising my time without packing 25 things into an hour. I used to be able to do that while spinning plates, changing nappies, cooking supper and doing a radio interview. I can't do that any more.

I don't need a lot of equipment or anything particularly fancy to work, but I did buy an ergonomic chair so I had somewhere comfortable to sit when I write. It's brilliant and I don't get backache any more. It was expensive, but it's important if you're sitting at a desk all day to make sure you're comfortable. The only other thing I need when writing is a kettle and teabags close by.

It's interesting how it takes our bodies a while to catch up with any life change. There was a point – and it's still the case to a small degree – when I couldn't do any work after four o'clock because that was when the children would come home from school.

With each book, I get through the process and at the end I'm glad it's done. But then the fear of sending my 'baby' out into a cruel and crowded world kicks in. The success of any book is all down to you, the reader, and I can't thank you enough for every book you've bought. The work is hard, but worth it and something good always comes out of the hard times. I guess, in a way, each new novel is a mini Repowering. And if I had allowed my imposter-syndrome doubts to stop me, I wouldn't have this amazing career now. When new opportunities come our way, we should grab them with both hands. Writing wasn't something I'd set my heart on – I didn't even know if I could write a book. But if I hadn't seized the opportunity when it was offered, I wouldn't have the reward I have now. It's more sedate than my previous career but that's OK, too.

Becoming a writer was a big part of my Repowering without even knowing it. If your Repowering involves changing career, starting up a side hustle or even a hobby, try to carve out a space in your home that's exclusively for this purpose. It doesn't need to be a whole room, maybe just a desk somewhere. The top of stairs and landings are often wasted space and can be a great location for a small desk.

We have a funny perception of writing here in the UK, which helps feed imposter syndrome. In America, anyone who puts pen to paper with the aim of maybe one day publishing it calls themselves a writer. Here, we fumble and apologise, not wanting to appear boastful or arrogant. It's the British way. But what I will say is, whether you are writing your journal, never to be seen by others, or pulling out a great novel from your own imagination, keep going. Just the act of writing can be a great way into your feelings.

Writing is such a personal thing. There's the fear of failing, the dread of a looming deadline and the terror that you will be exposed as an imposter. All that baggage acts like an anchor, holding you down. It's the same when we try to make changes in our personal lives. There's always something in the way. We think we'll work on ourselves once we've moved house or got that promotion. When the children are older, when we retire, when we've done that 10k run, or when ... or when ... or when ... The fact is, all these things are important, but we cannot let them keep us stuck in a rut. Sometimes we must meet ourselves where we are. Whatever our age, wherever we are on life's journey, the future begins now so we need to make sure we're squeezing the very last drop of joy out of it.

Believe me, I question almost everything I have ever done. Have I been a good enough mum? Is the new book going to sell or will someone find out I actually can't write? Am I really good enough to take my place in the room?

If you find yourself asking this last question, there is only one answer: of course you are, you absolute twit!

Putting Pen to Paper

Whether you're keeping a journal or attempting a novel, I'm a firm believer that writing things down helps to clarify your thoughts. Here are some of my tips for exercising your writing muscle.

- If you feel you have a book in you, then get going!
- Books are very personal. I'm telling you all sorts of embarrassing things I've done in this one. But those are the best bits!
- Take little breaks so that your brain doesn't get over-stimulated and grind to a halt. I always find a quick episode of *Frasier* or *Bargain Hunt* does the trick.
- Don't forget to go outside and breathe.
- And don't forget writing is REALLY hard and knackering ... or is it just me?

Chapter Five

Fern's DIY Guide to Boosting Self-Confidence

*T*o others, I look confident, but inside I'm often nursing low self-esteem. For instance, when *Strictly Come Dancing* came my way in 2012, I was unsure about how good I would be. My partner, a handsome Russian, was an incredible dancer but he would shoot from the hip. After we were partnered live on air, I found him sitting on the steps where the band play. I asked him if he was OK with having me as a partner and he said, 'Well, I am used to someone with some dance ability, and younger.' My confidence took a hit, but I laughed and told him that I didn't feel 55 and that, when I had a drink in me, I was a sensational dancer. He did not laugh. Rehearsals started and it was noted, by him, that I had no balance and couldn't dance, so I should just stand still while he danced around me.

Strictly is a magnificent sausage machine. You go in one end as a fairly normal person and come out the other as a bedazzling, spray-tanned, sequined goddess. I enjoyed the spray tans and the fittings for the incredible costumes. It was just the rehearsals that were challenging. As the weeks went on, I found it increasingly hard to gather up my self-confidence and there were days I was crying before I even got into the rehearsal room. My partner did sometimes get frustrated with me. One late evening, when I simply couldn't get the steps in my head and we were both tired, he looked at me and said, 'Go home before I kill you.' It was a joke. I laughed. 'Kill me, please.' I know this sounds grim, but it was funny too. At one point, I did start to worry I was suffering from Stockholm syndrome as I would do anything to try to please him. Finally, at the end of our journey, he said to me, 'Well, you did everything I asked of you.' Hearing that felt like I had received the glitterball.

So, did I grow in confidence during the gruelling experience? Well, the scores would probably indicate that I did. I lasted until week six, when we achieved our highest mark, dancing the salsa. I was wearing a fluffy, flouncy pink number which allowed ample freedom for my shimmies and my butt shakes. These costumes are built around a leotard, with a bra and microphone sewn in, so you are safe in the knowledge that they will never reveal things they shouldn't and everything is securely stowed away. That night, we scored 27 points, the most we'd ever achieved, before making an exit. When it's your time, it's your time, and I was prepared to leave the show in week six.

Then we went out on tour, where it was a different and better landscape. My partner and I had two dances with each other and there were a couple of group dances before the professionals took to the floor. As a couple, we danced the salsa and a Viennese waltz, which was my favourite. The pink outfit was out again for the salsa and, for the waltz, I wore a long, iron-grey chiffon dress that was swishy and smothered in Swarovski crystals, with a feather boa trim around the bottom; a nightmare for quick changes but a joy to behold. I never quite nailed the group dances but it was exhilarating to be in front of huge audiences. Performing at the O2 in front of 20,000 people, as well as other huge arenas plastered with giant screens during the five-week tour was an amazing experience.

There were two tour buses, one to transport the band between venues, and the other for the dancers and professionals. I started on the dancers' bus, where the air was thick with chatter about false eyelashes and heels. But I felt like an outsider and after a few days I asked if I could join the band on their bus instead. They laughed and welcomed me saying, 'We wondered how long it would be before you joined us.' What a different vibe! The musicians had fine wines and cheese and artisan bread for the journey. Ultimately, I came out of that entire episode relieved and feeling good. It was something of an endurance test but, in the end, it was great for bolstering my resilience ... and I survived! I used every TV trick in the book to lift myself up as well. A good spray tan, some sequins and a pair of false eyelashes and you end up thinking,

I'm pretty f**king good actually. At the end of the tour, I was gifted the dresses to keep. A most unusual honour! One day, they will be on display at the Fernywood Museum, the last thing you'll see before being pointed to the gift shop.

People often ask me if doing live television was nerve-wracking. I've done so much of it and there was a time when I was more often in a studio than I was at home. I used to joke about being more nervous opening my own front door than being in front of a camera.

Why did I feel so at home in a live studio? Was it just confidence or the feeling of being part of a big team where we each knew the part we had to play? Working in television, the lasting lesson has been not to dwell on myself too much. The yardstick that executives measure presenters by is relatability – they must be likeable. Beyond that, a presenter must be someone who realises they are not the star of the show. That role is reserved for the guest. On television, you talk to all sorts of people. One guest might be well versed in the media, such as an actress or politician, while the next might be wrestling with the aftermath of a monumental tragedy. In that case, the person sitting in front of you is utterly bereaved and battered. They have a story they want to tell and it's your job to give them the confidence to do so. It is important to be empathetic and listen, which makes them feel validated. After all, they find themselves in a place that's far from their comfort zone.

So, how is this going to help you when you're feeling nervous or lacking in confidence? My advice in a work
or social situation is to quietly give a bit of yourself to
everyone. Offer to make a tea or coffee, ask them about
themselves and listen to their answers. People will respond
to easiness. Then you'll think, *Well, perhaps I'm all right
after all,* and your confidence will grow. Someone once
said to me that nerves run like wildfire. This is particularly
true in a studio situation, but it's also true in life generally.
I've aways thought it's not my job to be nervous. My job
is to sit and listen to people, whether that's at work or
among friends.

As a teenager, my daughter Grace often used to get
anxious before a party. You'll probably recognise the symp-
toms: headache, feeling sick, a desire to stay at home? With
us both being great fans of Justin Timberlake, I would always
ask her, 'Hmm, what would JT do?' and she'd say, 'I don't
know,' and I'd say, 'He'd put his hat on and dance.' That
always made her laugh. I'm sure you can find a similar silly
image to lift you in those situations.

When it comes to Repowering, believe in yourself, trust
your instincts and let your confidence be the catalyst for
change. See, it's super easy. I'll pack up now and go to the
beach ... Seriously, though, it really is the case that you may
have to fake it until you make it. Even if you're feeling a bit
nervous, if you behave as if you're not, it will help.

I was told early on that, as a woman in TV, you must never show any sign of nerves. The person telling me this, a female presenter, went on to explain that if she even questioned a minor thing while on air, her male producer would instantly shift the next interview to her male counterpart. It's a good illustration of how tough women need to be in the workplace. Those old sexist rules – never cry in the office, say bold things in a quiet voice and work harder than any man – are as current as ever.

Women still have to work hard to be taken seriously, in television and elsewhere. Back in the eighties, nineties and noughties, women were expected to have an agile mind, while also looking magazine-shoot ready with perfect hair and elegant make-up. This wasn't the case for men. How wonderful, to be able to put on a suit and wear it every day for three months without so much as a comment from viewers. Even now, a lot of focus is still on what women are wearing, what's on their feet, how their face is made up and their hairstyle. It's the tunnel of fire we have to walk through.

I must admit, I didn't always like the clothes I wore in the studio. I was not in control of my appearance; it was more often down to what a boss liked or the stylist wanted, but you have to go with the flow. As far as I was concerned, my job was to concentrate on the interviews, not be hijacked by my appearance. Once I left the dressing room, I would not look in the mirror again. Even if I was about to interview the prime minister!

In fact, I've quizzed three prime ministers and one of them, Tony Blair, I interviewed three times. Against expectation, he wasn't always as confident as I supposed he would be. In 2009, for the BBC One series *Fern Britton Meets …* I went with the crew to his Grosvenor Square office. He arrived late, a bit pink in the face, having rushed after dropping his son at school. At first, his main concern was choosing the right tie, then he asked about make-up. We didn't provide make-up for interviewees, so he asked me if I had any powder or Touche Éclat (a useful cosmetic, which erases any undereye shadow). I handed him my powder compact and Touche Éclat, and he went off to his mirror to apply it. He did a pretty good job.

When the cameras started rolling, we talked about the Iraq war and a question suddenly popped into my head: 'If you had known then that there were no weapons of mass destruction, would you still have gone to war?' He replied, that yes, he would have done. I took a breath and thought, *Gosh, he's admitting something big because his previous argument had been that he* had *to go to war because Saddam Hussein had weapons of mass destruction …* Even though nobody could find them. Out of the corner of my eye I saw my director, whose face told me he had definitely said something controversial.

If you leave a pause in an interview, the interviewee will feel they have to fill it. So, Mr Blair continued with, 'Yes, I would still have thought it right to remove him [Saddam Hussein].' When the crew and I got out of there, we were all a bit stunned. The following day, perhaps wanting to thank him, I bought some powder, Touche Éclat, a comb and a small bag to hold them and delivered them to his office. I later received a handwritten note thanking me. Much later, at the Chilcot inquiry into the Iraq war, my interview with him was referenced and he admitted, 'After all these years of interviews, I've [still] got something to learn …' I do feel a certain compassion for him now because for the rest of his life he will have a security team surrounding him. He will never know the simple pleasure of strolling down to a café, sitting in the sunshine on his own and ordering a latte.

Before he got the top job, David Cameron came on *This Morning* to talk with a viewer about their shared experience of caring for a child with disabilities. His own son, Ivan, had a form of cerebral palsy and epilepsy. He empathised with her and revealed that his family had to jump over the same welfare system hurdles, acknowledging that even a man in his position as an MP and with money found it dispiriting.

Finally, Gordon Brown came on the show, and he was the loveliest man. He came to take phone calls from viewers worried about their pensions, savings and tax. One caller was so anxious about their financial situation that Mr Brown asked him to stay on the line, as he wanted to talk with him better after the programme. And he did. I don't know many MPs who would do that, let alone prime ministers. During his premiership he invited us to Number Ten, along with many others, for a Christmas bash. Winnie, who was a toddler at the time, had her picture taken by the tree outside and he showed us his office (with a banana on his desk). We also met his wife Sarah, who was delightful.

Again, I'm meandering off the subject. The thing is, lack of confidence can affect people starting out and those at the absolute top of their game. For today's celebrities, it is far worse, thanks to the presence of social media where comments about people are passed daily and in volume. It's a breeding ground for inferiority complexes that are triggered by the trolls, abusive keyboard warriors who like to stay hidden behind their screens. They have no life; their pettiness makes them feel powerful and we mustn't forget this. If it's the trolls who come for you, remember, they are not brave or courageous and not worth responding to, so don't.

Shoring up our confidence is important wherever we are in life. It might be that we want to make huge changes, we want to make some tiny tweaks or it could be that we're perfectly happy just as we are. The thing with life, though, is it's unpredictable. We have no idea what's around the corner, but whatever happens, it's undeniably true that we'll handle it more easily if we're firing on all cylinders.

We often need confidence in order to make changes in our lives. A sense of confidence and gut instinct can provide the fuel we need to propel ourselves towards our goals, whatever they may be. Confidence can embolden us to step outside our comfort zone and can underpin our determination for change. It will act as a guiding force and help you navigate any setbacks.

Repowering my own life has been, and continues to be, liberating. Mostly at ease with myself, I can say what I want and be who I want to be. A lot of this inner confidence comes with age. When you're 40, you learn to be able to say, 'No, I'm not going to do that.' When you're 50, you start to say, 'F**k off!' When you're in your sixties, you don't even have to say that.

These days I can protect myself better if somebody says something that in the past would have made me think, *Oh, is that aimed at me? Do you not like me? What have I done wrong? How should I change?* The truth is that some people will get you and some people won't.

Effective Repowering demands complete honesty with ourselves and it's a good moment to take stock of life. This doesn't need to be scary, but we do need to ask some tricky questions and be prepared to answer them honestly. Making lists is a good place to begin and it's great to start this in a positive way. Jotting down everything that makes you happy, that you're thankful for and that you want to explore more is a perfect way to begin. It makes you aware that you probably have an awful lot of things to be confident about already.

Then comes the slightly trickier bit – looking at all the bits of life you'd like to change. Sometimes the things we're unhappy about are relatively easy to fix with small changes in habits; at other times they seem so huge they feel just over-whelming. But that doesn't mean they can't be changed. Face your fears, and even if you're nervous about taking the first small step towards your goal, do it anyway. Each time you face a fear and overcome it, your confidence will grow.

Pay attention to how you talk to yourself and challenge that negative voice in your head if it pops up and says some-thing awful. Instead of focusing on everything that could go wrong, tell yourself how amazing it will feel if it all goes terribly right instead. And when it does go right, make sure you celebrate your achievements, however big or small, as this will motivate you to move on to bigger goals.

Remember, though, building confidence is a journey, and it takes time and effort. You will experience setbacks and confidence isn't linear – you may be self-assured at one time, less so at others. There will be times when people or events knock your stuffing out. Again, though, you have the power to pick yourself up. Be patient with yourself and celebrate your progress along the way.

Try to spend your time with people who elevate you. Great friends will rejoice for you when you succeed in something, just as you will for them. If Repowering for you involves a change in career, then look out for online groups of people who are already doing the job that you want. That's a great way to build a community and you get to both support others and be supported. Hopefully by meeting others in a similar position, you'll get to see that everyone has successes and failures, and good days and bad.

When cultivating confidence, it's important to remain realistic. Too much confidence might lead us to believe, 'That's it! I've cracked it!' Only for the next project to fall flat on its face and squash you with it. It's important to make sure we have balance in our wider life. Repowering is awesome, but any change in life can be tiring, so it's great to get the basics right and to make sure we're really taking care of ourselves as we explore new options. It also pays to have a good plan. By nature, I'm gung-ho, and that leads to a lot of false bravado. And that's how at 60-something I found myself touring in a stage musical.

When my agent first mentioned *Calendar Girls* to me in 2019, I said, 'Absolutely no.' Nothing could persuade me to do a musical. After all, I am not an actress. So that was that. I wasn't going to do it.

The following week, I got an email saying Gary Barlow, who had written the music for the show, wanted to have a coffee with me. I'd met him a few times when he was in Take That and I thought it was lovely to be invited, so I said yes. I had fully planned to tell him it was nuts to even think of casting me in such a role. I was going to drink the coffee, have a chat and give him a firm no. Then the meeting happened, and it wasn't just Gary and me and a takeaway latte. Somehow, I was in a room full of people with a script in my hand reading a scene in front of the writer, director, casting director and producer.

I remember looking around the wobbly-floored room of an 18th-century building in Soho and thinking, *Life doesn't get more bonkers than this.* Weirdly, they offered me the job and, perhaps even more inexplicably, I said yes. It had been a firm no and then it became a yes. I was flattered into it. It absolutely tested my confidence, and common sense, to breaking point.

I've tried acting once or twice, including in a couple of local pantomimes, because that's what you do! Those were hard enough, but also enjoyable. When I was doing *Calendar Girls*, I remember one day – my birthday – where we were in a hot rehearsal room in Kensington. The director said to me: 'I'm thinking of letting you go because you can read the script well sitting down, but you can't do it standing up …'

He means, I can't do acting, I thought to myself. So that was me, shredded in the second week of rehearsal and knowing there were eight months ahead on tour. Anyway, somehow I kept the job. He was right; I'm not a natural actress, but it was a tough way to find out. The cast were forgiving of my endless errors and I appreciated their support. I did try to get it right but there was one scene in which the director declared: 'It's just all too technical for you.' All I had to do was sit on a chair! It was difficult, but it was a big lesson in having to really own the mistakes you've made and to keep going. To dig deep. It was worth it in the end.

I made three good friends. One of them was the musical director Toby, who was visiting me when I first met Two Cups, and two fellow actresses also became pals. One is Pauline Daniels, a Liverpudlian stand-up comedian, who is both funny and an excellent singer. She was so good to me on tour, and we had such a great time. Then there was Rebecca Storm, a wonderful singer and actor who has done a lot of musicals and was a great lead. We became a little bunch. We'd share dressing rooms and laugh a lot.

Getting through a long tour is gruelling. One day we were in the dressing room complaining about there being two shows that day and I said, 'Well, we're here now.' There was a moment's silence and then we all fell about laughing. It became the catchphrase of the tour when anything got difficult. *Well, we're here now.*

I learned a lot about building myself back up after that catastrophic loss of self-esteem. So, firstly, identify your strengths: make a list of your skills, talents and accomplishments. Recognising what you're good at and reflecting on past successes can boost your self-esteem. As women we're not necessarily brilliant at patting ourselves on the back when we've done something well, but now is a time to do it.

It's easy to think we can work on our confidence and then it's fixed. Like changing a tyre. Of course, it's not nearly as simple as this. Human beings are messy creatures. We're a mass of contradictions. One day I might be glowing with confidence. The next I feel a complete fraud. The thing that always gets me through is the experience to know I WILL get through. Age and experience have gifted me enormous emotional strength. I believe you have that too, in spades.

Think of confidence as a workout. We don't expect to go to the gym once a week and then start running a marathon immediately. It all takes time and a little bit of grit until one day you find yourself enjoying it. Reconstructing confidence is like building muscle. We need to keep at it, constantly reminding ourselves bit by bit that we're good enough.

Fern's Essential Life List

What makes your life worth living? Write down the things you're grateful for and glance at the list every time you need a confidence boost. Here are mine:

- My marvellous, wonderful, gorgeous children.
- The great friendships with Boo and Two Cups.
- The cats, Lady Silky Paws, Barbara and Dr Iain Mackerel. The latter two are half-siblings from different fathers and were born just half a mile away in the village. When you're not feeling your best, cats will sit with you and wipe away your tears with their tails – or hold you at paw's length, depending on their mood.
- My home, which is very much a work in progress but is a place where I feel happy and safe.
- The great work opportunities that still come my way.
- The lovely response I get from readers of my books.

Chapter Six

Let's Get Physical

*H*ealth is wealth and we should never forget that. We get one body and it's our job to take care of it. I wish there was a magical, fun formula I could give you for staying healthy, but sadly it's not that exciting. We all know the rules and they really are worth trying to follow. In 2016, when I was fit as a flea, I had a hysterectomy and unfortunately developed post-op sepsis. The fact that I responded so well to treatment was because I was in such good shape. I had a resting heart rate of 50 beats per minute due to all the cycling, weight training and spinning classes I had been doing for years. I recovered well from the sepsis and was discharged from hospital after two weeks of intense antibiotics with a further op to drain the abscess in my abdomen. It took me two years to fully get my strength back, but I was grateful that I was alive.

During my Era of Indolence, I gained too much weight. A few years before, I had had surgery, on medical advice, to have a gastric band fitted. It helped me lose a lot of weight while exercising regularly and eating good, wholesome food. The band works by restricting the capacity of your stomach so that you don't overeat. However, in my Era of Indolence, not only did I stop exercising, I also stopped eating well. The irony of a gastric band is that it allows wine, chocolate, cakes and almost anything else full of sugar or fat to slip down very easily.

So, how did I get back on track? It was when I met the surgeon who was going to fix my shoulder. The operation is complicated and takes about four hours. If the surgeon was going to help me, I was going to help him by getting fitter in readiness for the op. I knew the waiting list was a year long so I had no excuse. Out went the cigarettes, and on went the running shoes. I became evangelistic about doing Couch to 5k (the NHS's running programme for beginners). The slow and steady approach is a great confidence builder and soon I was running just a few minutes more each time and my legs were getting stronger.

As for food? Well, we all know the rules, don't we? Protein in the form of eggs, cheese, yogurt, chicken, etc. to keep our ageing muscles strong. As many vegetables as you like (did you know broccoli is a good source of protein?), fruit and water.

I grew up with a sweet tooth but I am trying to master that by having a couple of satsumas or an ice lolly made with real orange juice whenever I have a craving for something sweet. They seem to do the trick.

I started eating properly again and this, coupled with the running, I think, meant that I once again found the feeling of satiety. The thing in your brain that tells you that you are full. I'd been first class at overriding that for quite a while.

The thing is, healthy eating is the cornerstone of well-being, providing our body with the essential nutrients it needs to function at its best. If we can manage to consume a balanced diet rich in fruits, vegetables, whole grains, lean proteins and healthy fats, while minimising processed foods, sugars and excessive salt, we'll be doing ourselves a real favour in the long term.

Couch to 5k is a fantastic concept and I'd recommend it to anyone because it starts slow, gradually building your confidence each week with totally achievable goals. For example, Week 1 eases you in gently with nothing longer than 7 x 60-second runs with 90-second walks in between to recover. The trick is to stick to the plan and not to get ahead of yourself, thinking you can skip over a week. You have to build yourself up gradually and you will amaze yourself that at the end you will be able to run for 30 minutes. It doesn't need to be fast; you don't even have to cover 5k. As long as you are running for 30 minutes nonstop after nine weeks of training, you graduate! I'm not intending to run a marathon or win any races, but it has changed how I feel and I really enjoy the fitness side of it. The free phone app is available via the National Health Service.

One of the aspects I love about running is that you get to do it outside, which I'm sure is good for the soul. I went for a run the other day, on a beautiful, unseasonably warm day. Spring in Cornwall is special. You feel it coming on when you are running because you are amongst it as it unfolds. It's the tiny details you notice. There's a wild herb called Alexanders, also known as horse parsley. It looks a bit like angelica, but the leaves are not as shiny. As it flourishes in coastal areas, its lime-green flowers are abundant in hedges, on cliffs and in sea walls across Cornwall between March and June. It was brought over by the Romans, who used it in cooking for its celery-like flavour, but now it's used as a botanical for some Cornish gins. It grows alongside bright yellow rapeseed blown in from the fields. As they die back, honeysuckle shoots and dog roses appear. I love these subtle changes in the palette, and even the blues of the sky and the whites of the clouds as the year progresses and the seasons change. It always lifts my mood as I run.

There's so much evidence about how moving every day can make an enormous difference to our physical and mental wellbeing. It doesn't have to be much and we don't have to push ourselves beyond our limits. If you're really not doing any exercise at all right now then just resolving to go for a walk every day can make a huge difference. About ten million people in this country suffer from arthritis and, with joint pain, it's tempting to retreat to an easy chair. But it's especially important for people who have arthritis to maintain a good exercise regime. This is because our bones need strong muscles for support and, if we don't exercise, it weakens those supporting muscles, which puts more stress on our joints. You don't have to go over the top and it's important not to overdo it, but keeping active is proven to reduce joint pain and increase bone strength, so it's worth doing. There are lots of helpful resources online where you can find out the best types of exercises for people with arthritis and you can also check in with your health provider for more information.

As someone who has arthritis myself, I try to practise what I preach and exercise regularly. It's an arbitrary number but if I hit 10,000 steps a day, I'm happy. Yesterday, it was 12,000 so that was good. I recommend getting a watch that can count your steps. It's motivating to have a Fitbit or something similar monitoring your daily activity. I keep a steps record on my phone and, if I don't have it with me for some reason, any steps I take feel wasted because I'm not getting closer to hitting that magic number! Whatever device you use can be inspiration enough to make you go the extra mile (or yard!). And you could set little challenges for yourself, like making sure you're averaging more steps than the week, month or year before. The app I use isn't overly complicated. I just want to know about the distance, the steps and the rate my heart is pumping. Those small wins, that's all I want. I don't want to be doing anything extreme, I don't even want to run with people – I like to just be on my own, doing my own thing – and it's good for my head, my body and my appetite.

I will often listen to something on the BBC Sounds app while I'm running. *Desert Island Discs* is the perfect run time. If you hate the idea of going solo, then maybe rope in a friend or join a running group. There are lots about, from ubiquitous parkruns through to smaller, more informal groups. How many steps have I managed today? Just 3,070 because I've been fretting about writing and, in doing so, only walking around the house.

Anyway, whether you run or do Pilates, whether you exercise alone or in a crowd, now is the point in your life where it is probably wise to recognise that you're worth the time. We're so good at putting the needs of others, and indeed the health of others, before our own that we some-times need reminding that we're important too.

If you want to go for a walk, a run or do some cold-water swimming, just do it. No one will judge what you look like in a swimsuit or care that you have to stop every few minutes when you first start. Remember what my mum would say: 'They're all too busy looking at themselves to be worried about looking at you.'

I do occasionally go cold-water swimming with Two Cups and a gang of girls (but never Boo! She's much too sensible). It's lovely doing it with a group and if it's a special occasion we hire out the sauna on the beach for afterwards. We are mostly in our sixties so if we can do it, so can you. Yes, the water can be freezing but you're in and out. Then it's hot coffee and home. It's both wonderful and grim all at the same time. Two Cups suggested I buy some wetsuit boots and wetsuit gloves, which has been a real game changer.

If you've always fancied cold-water swimming, then I encourage you to give it a go. It's absolutely acceptable to go in very slowly; you don't want to shock your heart if you're not used to it. Safety is critical so wear a brightly coloured warm hat to stay visible and if you're getting really keen, invest in an inflatable tow float that attaches to your ankle and will be pulled along in your wake (just in case someone needs to spot you). It sounds contrary but do a warm-up on the beach before heading into the waves, to get your muscles going. Also, it's better for beginners to keep their head above the water rather than dunking it down. Keep close to the shore and if you're swimming alone make sure there are lifeguards on the beach. I never swim on a beach without lifeguards, primarily because it's the sensible thing to do, but also because they're very easy on the eye. This appreciation clearly runs in the family because when my niece Rose was a teenager, she once dug deep holes outside the lifeguards' hut. When I asked what she was doing, she said she was setting a trap to try and catch one!

I did some wild swimming with Rose a few years ago and we shared a hilarious time. We went down to a secluded cove, took all our clothes off and swam naked, and it was the most liberating of things. There was nobody and nothing around … until we looked up at the cliffs and saw some walkers! So, we kept ourselves under the water for a bit longer than we initially planned. As we're both summer babies born into the Zodiac's Cancer sign, she and I were in our element.

Cold-water immersion is brilliant for both physical and mental wellbeing as, apparently, the shock of the cold water stimulates the release of endorphins, leading to a natural high and potentially reducing stress. Or you can ease yourself in gradually by turning the hot water down a bit when you are about to finish your shower, the Michael Mosley way. I've started doing this and it does give a spring in the step.

Cold-water swimming has become trendy. But funnily enough, I've been doing it since I was child on cold days at the beach; we just called it taking a dip back then! So, relive those childhood memories of getting into the water. You'll love it … eventually.

Cycling, too, has been a big thing for me. I've cycled all over the world – more of that later. If you fancy it, give it a go. There are few things as freeing as whizzing along a country lane on a bike. It takes you back to carefree teenage summer afternoons in a way nothing else can. If you live in a city and are nervous about the roads then I totally understand, but if you can find some quiet cycle lanes or parks you can ride through, it is worth it.

Now my shoulder is fixed, I'm going out on my proper road bike again. I have a few different bikes – none of them are lean racing bikes, but my hybrid road bike is my favourite and I've named him Sausage. I also have an electric bike, which is perfect for whizzing up hills effortlessly and also good for regaining your confidence on two wheels. It's also the ideal option if you're new to cycling or your fitness levels are a little low.

Often, we equate exercise with improving how we look, rather than how we feel. Yet I think exercising should be about achieving some kind of life balance. The fact is, even if we don't feel like it, getting out there and achieving that bit more than before will generally leave us feeling calmer, with our confidence boosted.

We all have one part of our body we dislike. Why not stop focusing on that and think about the bits you *do* like? For example, when I've got the right shoes on, I've got great ankles! If I tuck my boobs in and hoist the bra right up, I have a fantastic cleavage.

This isn't a fitness book, but the one thing I will say is it is much easier to cope with all that life throws you if you're feeling healthy. When you're in a lacklustre phase it is much more difficult to bounce back from any setback. This is as true of our brains as it is of our bodies. I'm beginning to see staying fit as one of our duties, not just to ourselves, but to the NHS and our families. It's rarely ever too late to start doing more to improve the way you are, right now.

There are many ways to keep your brain sharp and that is also never too early to start. Smartphones are much maligned for the constant availability of social media and news, but they also have benefits, such as a great library of mental puzzles. I love them. My morning routine is this: I get up, feed the cats and then go back to bed with a cup of tea. I open up my phone and look through the BBC News headlines before diving into the puzzles. I start with Wordle, then an easy crossword, maybe Sudoku, a Codeword and Connections. If I get them all right, the feeling of satisfaction adds a little swagger to my day.

Our poor brains have taken a lot of information in over the years. I am at the point where I think most of my brain storage is full. It's not so easy to retrieve answers when I'm watching *Pointless* or *The Chase*. I'm even having to double-check my spelling nowadays and I have always been a good speller. Am I losing some of my sharpness? Mind you, I never have been able to keep up with all the children's and all the pets' names. It's so irritating!

When I was younger, I'd put something down and, even though I hadn't really registered it, I knew where it was.

Now, I struggle to find everything. At my age you periodically see the doctor and say, 'Am I losing my marbles because half the time I can't remember why I've gone upstairs?'

'No, no, you're fine,' they'll say. 'You really are fine. You know who the prime minister is?'

'Yes,' I'll reply. 'It's Gladstone, I think ...'

It's not just age that does this, it's also stress. If you've got too much going on in life, try to stop ruminating and allow your head to empty a little and do some daydreaming. Sit quietly with no distractions and ease your thoughts into quietness. Relax. Notice your breath and if you want, try to slow it down. I learnt a bit of this in lockdown online yoga sessions, which were so soothing. If you can focus your brain on your breathing, the intrusive thoughts are less likely to pop in. Try it for a few minutes each day.

If you're lucky enough to have a child or grandchild with you, play a game of checkers (aka draughts) with them. Such a simple game and yet utterly fiendish. I play with Winnie and she hammers me every time, but it keeps my brain alert! Learning something new, such as a language or a musical instrument, is a great way to get the brain working. (My fantasy is to fly off to Italy for a year and learn to speak the language – maybe one day!) Anything new we learn, even if it's from something as simple as taking up a new hobby, can help our brains adapt and change, which is important at any age. All these are just suggestions. You will find your own.

Friends keep you sane, too. Last time I got together with Boo and Two Cups, we had enormous fun just chatting about life. We were sitting in Two Cups' beautiful conservatory, named Petersham after Petersham Nurseries in Richmond, London. (Check them out online and you'll see how gorgeous it is.) Two Cups and her husband are adorably eccentric and love all things cowboy and country and western. So she has bought herself a lariat, which to the uninitiated is a lasso, and she has been practising with it. It's a second-hand one and she says it's great because it's been greased by the palms of sweaty cowboys.

We were chatting about our health and how we enjoy having the last meal of the day earlier and earlier. My stepmother mocks me for wanting a 5pm supper. She always says, '*How* early?' That's nursery tea!' But Boo and I get terrible reflux and if we eat after 5pm we can't sleep! Two Cups then began moaning about how young the doctors are and how they don't listen to her now that she's a woman of a certain age. (On the subject of doctors, she's rather keen to move to the Scilly Isles but feels it's too much of a risk because if she had an emergency she'd have to be helicoptered off to the mainland.) We sat and contemplated the terrible truth that all doctors, policemen and teachers look to us like children, then she turned to her lovely husband: 'Get me more bubbles – I can't get up because my knees hurt.' Apparently, she's going to get them fixed by going on a machine that grows new cartilage in just two sessions. Boo and I told her we didn't believe this could possibly be true.

Boo is one of the most level-headed women I know. She has made a gorgeous, welcoming home that we absolutely love visiting. You know the cottage in the film *The Holiday*? It has that vibe. She's a wonderful host and manages to squeeze lots of us around her table while feeding us incredible food. She also makes a great Cosmo! Most importantly of all, she is my absolute social linchpin. If she hadn't said hello to me at the village dog show, our lovely friendship might never have happened. I'm so grateful she did. I love her even more because that night in Petersham she suddenly said, 'I wish I had told a lot more people over the years to f*ck off.' We all drank a toast to that.

As the bubbles flowed, Two Cups started telling us about a local book club. Apparently, the book under discussion was *Untamed* by Glennon Doyle, about a woman on a journey of self-discovery. The book club readers all agreed they hated it, mainly because they thought it only appealed to younger women. But in a nod to modern society, someone had made chocolate cake laced with cannabis – hash brownies, if you will. It wasn't long before there was perpetual laughter and then they all got the munchies and had to have half a packet of chocolate digestives and two rounds of toast each. Apparently, everyone slept like logs that night. The women of this book club prove my point, that it's important not to be afraid of change. While I am definitely not endorsing the use of recreational drugs, having a change is good, healthy and sometimes unavoidable.

I told you I took up smoking as a late-in-life hobby, but I haven't told you how I finally gave it up. The story begins on a night out with my niece Rose and her friend Lil, at the local church hall, where a wonderful comedian called Johnny Cowling was doing his show. He's brilliant, by the way. Anyhow, his first act was exceptionally funny and then there was a brief break so everyone could get a beer and a pasty. I went outside for some air and ran into a friend. She was smoking and, while I had been trying very hard to cut down, I asked if I might have one. I really enjoyed it. Then we went back in for the second half of the show, which comprised Johnny singing Elvis songs with his talented wife Sarah providing the music, and we all got up and danced. As the night came to a close and we left the hall, we were all grateful for the cool night air after the heat and sweat of having a good time.

As I drove out of the car park, I saw the girl who'd 'lent' me the fag and asked if she'd give me another to drive home with. So, there I am driving home, fag on, when suddenly that colossal nicotine hit that makes you want to throw up washed over me. I was getting close to home and drove down the lane trying very hard not to be sick, but a wave of nausea hit hard, so I stopped the car and stood on the edge of a field retching into a hedge. I was bending over to be sick and the force of the retching caused me to fart really loudly! Rose and Lil had the windows down and of course heard everything. They erupted with laughter and said, 'Classy lady' over and again in sing-song voices. And that, dear reader, was the day I gave up smoking. I've said no to any cigarette offered ever since.

It's very hard to go from being unfit to being more active, so don't over-stretch yourself. The important bit is not to quit. I find writing hard so I know how it feels. You just have to start doing a little and a little and a little. If you're doing press-ups, for example, you might only manage three, but that's OK. Make the three as good as you can and then next time you train, see if you can add another one. Caring for ourselves means eating well, exercising regularly, getting good quality sleep (and enough of it) and taking time out to relax. These are big goals to dangle in front of you but I'm all about increments. Stick with it and small steps will soon turn into mighty strides.

Feel the Burn with Fern

- Download the Couch to 5k app on your phone, as a surefire way to start or resume a running regime.
- If you honestly feel you can't run, try walking.
- Do planks daily to improve core strength.
- Eat protein.
- Share the ins and outs of ailments with friends and have a laugh while you are doing so.
- Exercise your mind as well as your body.

Chapter Seven

All About You

*W*hen you listen to the safety announcement on a plane, the flight attendant clearly tells you that, in the event of a loss of cabin pressure, you must put your own oxygen mask on first before helping other people, even children. If you don't then you are at risk of not being able to help anyone at all. Well, this is as true on the ground as it is at 35,000 feet. If we don't pay attention to our own immediate needs, then we will eventually burn out, rendering ourselves useless in caring for everyone else.

If you imagine love and care as a cash budget, it's easy to see how much we splurge on our children, partners, colleagues, friends, cats, dogs and acquaintances and leave ourselves with just enough to scrape by. This isn't OK. We also deserve attention and care. I think it's possible and hugely desirable to learn to redirect all the caring skills we've used on others over the years and spend some on ourselves. We deserve it.

This might sound selfish to you at first, but let me introduce you to a new word – self-ist. The difference is subtle but, once I began to explore it more, it made perfect sense.

Being selfish means mainly putting yourself first regardless of the impact this might have on others. Being selfless means you do the opposite and put the needs of everyone else before your own. A more self-ist approach means making better choices for your own wellbeing.

To be self-ist is to have an awareness of the situations, obligations and responsibilities that are doing you no good at all. Sometimes you just have to honour your own needs and wishes while also being mindful of the consequences for others. This is a great philosophy because it means you don't automatically give away any power and end up doing something that is draining and could leave you feeling resentful.

We all need to love and be loved in return. It's a basic human need. It is precious and should be nurtured at all costs. The love of friends enriches our souls. The love of children sustains us and don't get me started on the love I feel for my cats! Love for life partners is different again.

I was married all the way through my thirties, forties, fifties and early sixties. So, I had 30 years of being a wife to two husbands. You'd think it would have been tricky to slip back into single life after such a long time, but it is much easier being on my own now than it was in my twenties. Back then, I remember being single for a year or so, and feeling as if I was on the shelf. I was rash about relationships when I was younger and would rush into them. Perhaps if I knew then what I know now (put that on a T-shirt!), I wouldn't have been in so much of a hurry.

I have found being single liberating. I didn't expect to be single in my sixties but I have friends. I have a social life. I can spend a lot of time in my pyjamas round the house, which is heavenly. I'm perfectly happy most of the time. There are many positives, chief among them being the sheer freedom of making decisions entirely for myself (rightly or wrongly). I love being my own person and having my own agency. Being able to choose what I want for supper, whether I go to bed at six o'clock in the evening or two o'clock the next morning. I'm not saying it's been easy for me all the time – but I'm making it work.

My days now are pretty perfect. Sometimes, I'll decide to work on the next book for a few hours and then take a walk around the garden or nip over to Boo's and have a cuppa. If it's sunny and I've done enough work, I'll get in the car and drive to the beach. The other night, I went down there and took a bottle of zero-alcohol beer with me to drink sitting in the dunes, people-watching. There were families and young couples and handsome lifeguards running up and down the shoreline. My life, my choice.

As women, we take on the mental load and emotional labour on behalf of our families, friends and colleagues.

More often than not, it becomes our obligation to write the Christmas cards, make sure the fridge is stocked, see that the cats have had their jabs or that the dog has had a pee and, to top it off, source thoughtful, exquisite presents for in-laws.

We take on so much and often it's not even ours to take on. I like men very much. I enjoy their company, humour and conversation, but I do question how some fully grown men find it so hard to buy their mum a birthday present or put on a load of washing. I know they're not all like that by any means, but you do hear some stories …

Take holiday packing, for example. Women meticulously fill a case with everything we might need while our partner says, 'I only need my shorts.' Then, once we're on holiday, he'll say, 'Have you got some toothpaste?' or 'Did you pack a razor?' Come on, lads. Your wife/girlfriend is not your mum. Husbands should pack for themselves. Nobody else should do it for you.

Why do some women think their man needs to be molly-coddled? Are we closet masochists? Or, more close to the truth, is it because we need that sense of control? If that's the case, well, it's probably because we feel it's not going to get done otherwise. Then we start behaving like a sighing martyr and everyone is left feeling grumpy. Sometimes we can be our own worst enemies. I'm a positive person and Repowering is all about optimism and open-mindedness.

But there's always an exception to prove the rule, and here it is. We have got to the embrace the power of saying 'no'. Try it. It's wonderful. No, no, no, no, no. Even the most meek and mild nuns have to learn to say no sometimes; a nun told me that herself.

Saying no can feel hard and alien at first but keep practising and you'll find, like running, it gets easier. It's a powerful tool in your self-care armoury.

We really can't Repower effectively until we have learned to say no. It can be hard but it's such an important skill to learn. Of course, we worry about conflict, feel guilty, are anxious about rejection or disapproval and often have an over-developed sense of duty. All of that is natural. We're nice people, we like to help out, we don't want to let others down, and, as women, we have been taught from a young age that it is our job to please other people.

This is where boundaries come in – and I am literally the worst person to talk about this. I find it difficult to set boundaries when it comes to information about myself. I am too open. I have few secrets left. But I am learning to say no and it is a game-changer. It's amazing that such a simple word can make such a huge difference to your life. It saves you time and energy, freeing you to focus on things that really matter to you. It's almost as if you're giving yourself extra hours in the day. And the person who is receiving your 'no' will begin to understand your boundaries better.

Each time you say yes to something you don't want to do, you're just adding another thing to your schedule, and we all know that being too busy can leave us feeling frazzled. Or, perhaps worse, we drop something we'd love to do in favour of the more tedious thing. Either way, if we'd just been able to say no in the first place, life would feel that bit better.

The children are always telling me about Netflix stuff that I will never watch, or TikTok clips when I'm not even on blooming TikTok, or books that I will never read. Learning to say no to these unwanted recommendations has been wonderful; I'm not watching or reading stuff that doesn't interest me. I'm just too old and uninterested to be doing with any of it and I don't have that sort of time left. And also, please don't send me a voice note. Yes, it may be quicker for you, but it is flaming dull for me to use precious moments from my life listening to you telling me you've missed your train.

Standing up for yourself and clearly stating your needs is a key to Repowering. Each 'no' you say is a reminder that your time, feelings and priorities are important. It's one of the simplest ways to give your power an extra boost. I know what I want to watch and read and being able to say no to other things means I'm not stretched too thinly. I have the time and the desire to do the things I like. You will find that you start to use your nos and yeses more wisely and to greater effect. Think about that when you keep getting more work piled on you with ever-tighter deadlines. Something has to give and these are never good circumstances to give our very best. Simply say, 'That's very kind of you but I am not the best person for that. Mr/Ms X is much better suited.'

When we set our boundaries it's important to be clear, honest and direct. A simple, 'I can't do this right now,' or 'That's awfully kind but I won't be able to make it,' are much better than endless waffling and excuses. Never lie when you say no, as you will invariably forget the lie or spend way too much time and energy inventing a second cousin and their marvellous wedding that you just couldn't miss to sidestep a tricky dinner party!

When you start to say no, you'll find you have more time, so why not ringfence some of it just for you? Use it to think about what your future might be like. Fantasise about it – you can always come back to reality a bit later. If you just begin thinking about things, it gives you hope and allows you to explore how you'd like your life to look. That's the start of Repowering.

Often a single incident can lead us into life changes. Your last child goes off to uni. The family dog dies. You lose a job you love. The need to Repower becomes obvious and compelling. Sometimes, though, it isn't like that; it's more a restless kind of feeling that leads us to believe there's something better for us out there somewhere, which can lead to resentment if you don't act on it. It will eat you up inside if you're not careful.

We all endured the Covid pandemic. It was a time of collective trauma and for most of us they were a couple of dark years. The horror of so many deaths and the grief that subsequently spread through families here and elsewhere across the globe moved us all. Many of us became unwell. It left us, if not depleted, then certainly changed. I was lucky that I didn't lose anyone to this awful disease and have a sense of guilt that, in the face of national jeopardy, I was somehow let off the hook. You might feel the same.

In the early days, I'd sit out in the garden and the silence was extraordinary, wasn't it? There was no air traffic. Not even a tractor in the lanes. And for the first time in a long time, we were all aware of the birdsong, sounding louder than ever before. We could walk on the beach or go out on bikes as long as we stuck within our radiuses and our bubbles. It was so peaceful, but it was also transformative for me.

Some months before, my then husband came down to Cornwall and we sat at the kitchen table and had *the discussion*. We had reached the end of a shared road. Our dual carriageway was reducing to single lanes. Life as a couple had been wonderful, exciting, fulfilling, and we'd shared many happy times. He brought a lot into my life and I brought a lot into his. But when it's over, it's over. I got through it all, I think, by looking forward, not seeing only what was right under my nose but looking beyond and thinking, *It'll be fine by next week, next month, next year.* It might not be the best way, but it's the only way I could do it. I am a great believer in putting one foot in front of another and repeat. I hear my mum's voice telling me, 'This too will pass.' So, I just focused on what was ahead. In general, I rarely look back. I just keep going.

One thing is certain, though: if you're reading this, you got through difficult times, too. Probably with wounds and hurts, but you made it. And that's what we have in common. We coped. We're here now. We're on the other side and it's our duty to find out who we are and to get back to life.

Humour me for a moment. What is your dream? How would you change your life to make it more exciting or fulfilling? Where would you be and who would you be with? Imagination is such a powerful thing. I remember how my mum, even as an adult, liked to play pretend, inventing fantasy lives to entertain herself. I was on holiday with her once and I overheard her saying to someone, 'Oh yes, I'm an upholsterer, I specialise in antique furniture.' She didn't, but she let her imagination do the talking and it opened up a hilarious conversation, which amused us both. I think perhaps it's a family trait because her mother, my grandmother, was also prone to a tall tale. I remember the days when children were allowed to go and buy cigarettes and I was off getting her 20 Kensitas at the local paper shop. The man behind the counter asked me if they were for my grandmother. I said they were and he replied: 'Isn't she wonderful for 80? Isn't she great? She looks amazing.' My grandmother was in her sixties at the time. Isn't *that* great?

My daughters and I are excellent at talking nonsense. We improvise long and convoluted, often hilarious stories that amuse us for hours. We each have highly tuned imaginations and make up characters that we find very entertaining. I'm not sure any of it would translate very well if seen or heard by an audience but the pure silliness of it is enough to really cheer us up.

My father invented a character called Mr William who is a heavenly weather forecaster. If, for example, we really needed good weather for an event or a trip, my father would say, 'I've had a word with Mr William.' Mr William was rather Victorian. He had a winged collar and stood at one of those tall desks, no seat, with a ledger and a quill pen. My father would say, 'Mr William, could you make sure that the second of May is good for me?' Mr William would turn the pages and say, 'Hmm, the second of May? I'll do my best,' and scratch a note with his quill. Mr William always came through.

Mr William wasn't the only 'guiding spirit' in our family. Have you discovered the parking angel, Saint Philomena? She is marvellous and 99 per cent of the time she'll find you a space. You have to give her at least a 15-minute warning, and be super polite. I might say: 'Saint Philomena, if there's a chance of a parking space I would love one but I understand if someone else needs it more than me.' And blow me, I get there and there's a space. I mean, pretty much always. Even somewhere that's usually incredibly busy. I don't know where these things come from and, of course, it's all claptrap. Or is it ... ?

Many people swear by manifestation, which is really a more formal way of imagining your dream life. People say it works. You can write down, *I'd like a blue Porsche for my birthday, please. Oh, and I want my company to be turning over £2 million by next July.* And they will tell you it worked.

I'd ask for simple things like, *Can I find an electrician who can stop the lights in the bathroom flashing on and off because doing my make-up in a strobing disco is driving me mad?* It hasn't worked. Perhaps it only works for big things. So far, it hasn't worked for me but then I don't believe it's all about the flashy motors and rolling in money.

The reason it's interesting in the context of Repowering is not necessarily because the universe is going to deliver. It's more that, if you write down your goal and behave in a way that supports it, you are much more likely to create the life you really want. If I wrote down, *I want an electrician,* but then rang everyone I knew who might know one, the chances are I'd be lucky. I guess it's just spurring you on to do your own spadework.

It's like the parable of the drowning man that's often told as a joke. You know the one. Picture the scene … a quaint little town nestled in the rolling hills, where the people gather in a charming church to seek solace from life's trials. But, lo and behold, trouble brews as dark clouds gather and rain pours down, turning streets into rivers.

In the midst of this tempest, there's a vicar, a man of unwavering faith. He's kneeling on the church porch, his heart lifted in prayer. As the floodwaters inch higher, a kind soul paddles by in a canoe, urging him to flee to safety.

'Come, Vicar,' they implore. 'The waters are rising fast.'

But our steadfast vicar, bless his soul, refuses, trusting in the divine hand to guide him. As the situation grows dire, a rescuer arrives in a motorboat, shouting urgent warnings of impending disaster. Yet still, our vicar remains resolute, convinced that his faith will see him through.

Alas, as the levee breaks and chaos reigns, only the church steeple stands defiant above the raging waters. Our vicar is clinging on to it, a beacon of faith in the storm. Then, from the heavens themselves, a helicopter descends, offering salvation.

'Take the ladder, Vicar,' the rescuer implores. 'This is your last chance.'

But even then, steadfast in his belief, the vicar refuses to let go of his trust in the divine plan. And so, tragically, he meets his end in the floodwaters. Yet, in his righteousness, he ascends to the gates of heaven, seeking answers from the Almighty.

'Lord,' he pleads. 'I trusted in you completely. Why did you not save me from the flood?'

And, with a gentle shake of His head, God replies: 'My dear child, I sent you not one but two boats and even a helicopter. What more could you have asked for?'

This is useful to consider in the context of manifestation. Just writing down a shopping list of luxury cars, foreign cruises and elusive electricians is never going to work. Whereas clearly defining what you want, changing your behaviour to make your goal more attainable, recognising lucky breaks and accepting help when it's on offer is a sure-fire recipe for success.

I think manifesting can be helpful in that it allows us to explore our subconscious in a safe and creative way, particularly if we're not sure where we're going next. Proponents of manifestation recommend putting together a mood board of images that inspire you. If you do this and one of the pictures you stick on it is a house by the sea, then perhaps your subconscious is telling you that maybe you want to move to the seaside. Or if it's a minimalist loft in a metropolis, perhaps you are being told that deep down you yearn for big city life. Or maybe it's just telling you that you should do a bit of decluttering!

I guess where manifestation differs from simply making a plan and sticking to it comes down to having a belief in something bigger than ourselves. I'm quite pragmatic about life. I know I'm determined enough to make what's in front of me work. I don't often project into the future. I think about tomorrow and next week and that's about as far as I can go, but I am a great list-maker. So, if list-making is like manifesting, then I'm all for it.

Sometimes the universe delivers in strange ways. I had always wanted to come down here to Cornwall to live full time and it happened. It was an unfortunate set of circumstances that got me here, but here I am and I absolutely, wholeheartedly know it is where I am meant to be.

While manifesting might sound a bit out there, it's grounded in sound principles from psychology, neuroscience and even quantum physics. At its core, manifestation is the belief that our thoughts and emotions have a direct impact on our reality. From a psychological standpoint, the practice aligns perfectly with therapies such as CBT (cognitive behavioural therapy), which teaches you to shape your behaviour and outcomes by reframing your thoughts and using visualisation.

Neuroscientists suggest that our thoughts are powerful enough to help fashion certain patterns of thinking and perception. Quite simply, this means if we think we can, we can – and if we think we can't, we can't.

As for quantum physics, it's all way too complicated for me, but one facet of it implies our intentions can influence the behaviour of particles, suggesting a connection between consciousness and the physical world.

So, there you have it. There's an awful lot of science behind my advice to sit quietly and have a little think about exactly what it is you want from the rest of your life. It's obviously a bit of a cliché, but today really is the first day of the rest of your life …

Futureproof with Fern

The sands are slipping through our timer. Make the most of every moment.

- Don't waste time watching a film that's under par.
- You don't have to finish every book you start. If you aren't enjoying it, snap it shut and give it away to someone who might.
- Leave a play at the interval if it's not for you.
- Don't be fooled into ordering poached eggs on sourdough. Sourdough is not user-friendly to our older, tender mouths and teeth!
- Finally, if you like to cling film leftovers for tomorrow but hate the fight with the cling film box, I highly recommend getting a Wrapmaster 1000. You'll thank me for it.

Chapter Eight

Love Me Tender, Love Me True

(Part 1)

*A*s a child I loved fairy tales and didn't we all buy into the whole Cinderella dream? I read it to my sons and my girls and I'll read it to my grandchildren if I have any, because it's a delightful, powerful story of love.

But it is just a story.

Projecting into her future, poor old Cinderella will still have to invite those bloody sisters and her evil stepmother to the castle for tea and they'll be wandering around, checking for dust and being rude to the servants. And the prince will suddenly be, 'Oh, I've got to see a man about a dog,' and he'll piss off and she'll be left to do everything. That is the reality. Do they live happily ever after? I doubt it.

For Cinderella, finding her prince was relatively clear-cut, once her fairy godmother appeared and waved her magic wand. There's nothing straightforward for the rest of us. I find the idea of embarking on a new relationship terrifying and tempting in equal measure. What frightens me? Mainly the idea of losing my independence.

However, I was talking to a friend recently and she reminded me that being in a relationship doesn't necessarily mean giving up your independence. This notion came as a surprise and is something I need to process before I fully comprehend it. My behavioural pattern has always been to give away my autonomy in a relationship. I realise that I did this because I was brought up to be obedient and why wouldn't I want to share everything? Including my own agency? My power?

I can now think more about the joy that meeting someone might bring into my life, while keeping the best bits of my new single existence. I imagine what it would be like to have a voice on the end of the phone. Someone to talk to and walk with. Someone with whom to share hobbies, hold hands and maybe ... gulp ... get intimate. While I'm open to the possibilities, I'm also frightened because I don't want to make myself unhappy again. It's painful for everyone. So, why would I want to have another gamble on love? That sounds a bit bleak, I know, so it may make you laugh to hear that I recently wrote a little list of the kind of person I'd like to meet. Top of the list was someone who is creative, kind, enjoys reading, can laugh, is kind, honest, a gardener, a friend, and did I mention kind? Do you have anyone in mind? I know there are tons of lovely, uncomplicated men out there ...

It's daunting at any stage of life to get naked with someone new. These days my body looks as if it could do with a good iron or perhaps even better a steam press. So that's a whole added layer of pressure. I have wrinkles, wobbly thighs and bosoms that I roll up like a Swiss roll to tuck them in my bra. (By the way, if Mr Right is reading this, that's a joke!) Could I display all this to a new partner? I genuinely don't know but I will keep you informed.

It's not just my body I'm worried about sharing, mostly it's my personal space. I'm enjoying decorating the house the way I want to, designing a garden so it is how I like it, driving a car of my choice and wearing clothes that take my fancy. I love being in control of what I watch on TV, with no one snatching the remote from me. It is absolute heaven. Of course, these things don't necessarily have to stop when you're in a relationship, but I would have to consider a new partner's feelings and perhaps make some compromises. Possibly ...

What I would really like is a semi-detached relationship. One where we live in our own houses and not in each other's pockets. It would be lovely to ring this mystery man up and say, 'Would you like to come over for lunch?' or 'Have you got the name of a good plumber?' And he would probably ask me similar things. I'd like someone I can talk to about theatre, books and film, while walking on the beach with a pasty.

I'm chatting away about an imaginary fella, but where would I even meet one? I mean, I haven't been on a date since I was 26. I know people swear by internet dating, but it's not something I could do. If the press found me on a dating app I would be torn to shreds.

Dating is great – so I'm told – after you take time to reflect on previous relationships and look hard at what went wrong, what worked and what didn't. I'm now aware that I need to really know myself before I even think about heading out on a date. I must drop the emotional baggage. No date wants to hear about everything that's previously gone wrong in your love life. That's what girl-friends are for!

Repowering is a great time to take stock, to take a hard look at your previous romance CV and be brutally honest. What things do you repeat and where can you do better? If you're fresh out of a relationship, ask yourself if you're ready to dive back into dating – some time alone might just be exactly what you need right now.

You may even decide on a bit of a makeover. Why not? A splurge on your wardrobe and your make-up. Maybe a new pair of earrings? I'm all for it. The one thing I urge you not to do is to cut your hair. There is a thing called the f**k-it factor. A moment when you throw caution to the wind, go mad and do something that isn't easily reversible. Agreeing to a dramatic new haircut is one of those things. Wait until your emotions have settled and be absolutely certain before taking that particular plunge. It'll save you a lot on tissues. I am speaking from experience here ...

Largely, thoughts of romance and where it would fit in my life do not loom large in my everyday thinking. But occasionally on your Repowering journey they probably will pop into your head. Proceed with caution. Only you know if you have processed your past and are ready. Although sometimes I like the idea of meeting someone, I know in my heart I'm still not ready for a relationship. Scared? Yes. Interested? Yes. Ready? No.

With age and experience, I'm also more aware of what *I* have to offer in a relationship, both good and bad. I hope I am an easy-going person. I'm kind, thoughtful and caring. I don't need millions spent on me. I can be fun and be a bore. I can irritate and annoy. Be dull, impulsive, funny and emotional. There are times when, if I'm pushed far enough, I will suddenly erupt. In short, I am human.

Another reason I am wary of entering into a relationship is because I don't want to make anyone unhappy, and I don't want to be unhappy. Often, we blame the person we're married to rather than looking at what we could do differently next time. I was married to two fine men. I need to take some more time alone to think hard about my hopes and desires. For now, the great thing is I've realised I don't need to struggle with worrying about meeting someone right now because I'm happy working on myself and making my single life the best it can be.

I wouldn't have a clue how to behave on a date anyway. The last time I went on one was in the 1980s. Dating back then was incredibly different to how it seems now. For one thing, you would have to wait for someone to ring you up and ask you out. Now people just seem to swipe on their phones and a date magically appears. Dating was fun back then and so exciting. I met some intriguing people. Some who were skint. Some who had a bob or two (not that it makes a difference at all). It did mean I went on some varied dates. Many of them made me laugh so much that I can remember them very fondly.

Dressing up for dates was such fun too. At that time, I got a lot of my clothes from the Next catalogue as it had just arrived on the fashion scene. It was revolutionary. Each page had fabric swatches, so you could see and feel exactly what it would be like. (Don't judge me, this was the eighties!)

I remember one date with a boyfriend when I wore white leather trousers and a bluebell-coloured jumper that was very soft, both from Next. He took me to a local Chinese in Southampton. Over sweet and sour chicken, crispy chilli beef and egg fried rice (with me trying to make the chopsticks work), he turned to me and said: 'I really like what you wear because it doesn't annoy me.' That might sound strange to you but I laughed and took it as the compliment it was meant as, because he had noticed what I was wearing and made a nice comment. I liked him tremendously and we saw a lot of each other, eventually parting as friends.

Back then, boyfriends just seemed to turn up out of nowhere. People I didn't even know would ask me out. It was the way things worked. It was such fun not knowing what, or who, would turn up next. And a romance would often start not with a date but a kiss. I vividly remember being in a local pub in Cornwall when I was in my early twenties. I bumped into a man I knew in passing and we got chatting. I suspect we'd both had a couple of drinks because suddenly we were kissing and it was electric. He was great. I flattened a lot of grass with him. In fact, he was the one who came up with the phrase in the first place.

Then there were the parties. Walking into a room full of strangers was thrilling. It's a different story now and the mere thought of a party excites, terrifies and bores me in one. I was a different person back then and that's one of the reasons I'm so committed to Repowering now. The point is that back then I was carefree and unburdened, and that is the person I want to find again. I know she's still in me. She can still make me laugh. But the me I am now has decades of experience and can perhaps guide her a little better.

We don't talk a lot in our culture about platonic friendships but they can be just as fulfilling and supportive as romantic relationships. I wonder if my friendship with Boo and Two Cups would be the same if I were not single. I don't know. But if I ever do meet a new partner, it will have to be someone they've scrutinised first.

In all areas of your life, it's important to 'let the right ones in'. People often fall into one of two categories – fountains or drains. Fountains are those delightful souls who radiate positivity and energy and you are always glad to see them. Drains are the ones who sap your energy. They're quick to highlight problems, often leaving others feeling deflated and stressed. Recognising these two traits can help us to surround ourselves with fountains, those wonderful people who make life brighter, while learning to gently disengage the drains.

There's a quote above my desk by Maya Angelou: *When someone shows you who they are, believe them the first time.* When I first heard this it really struck me at my core. I don't want to generalise, but I know many women who've made excuses for people – often men – who have behaved badly. We all tell ourselves things such as, perhaps he's had a bad day, or a difficult childhood, or his boss has been mean to him, his car has broken down or whatever. But in inventing these excuses for others we are doing ourselves a great disservice.

If we get a bad feeling about someone, we should absolutely listen to our inner voice. In situations like these it's there to protect us. If the person in front of us is making us feel uncomfortable, then we need to heed that feeling. It's never a good idea to think that with a bit of kindness from us they will become a different person. If we went shopping for a van, we would never go into a Mini dealership, pick the smallest model and expect it to grow to meet our needs. It is the same with people. Sure, with the right motivation and with a lot of soul-searching someone can change themselves, but this is their job and not yours.

Is your relationship robust enough to bear a difficult conversation? Or would you rather put it off? You may want to say, 'We've got this far, I don't dislike you, though I am a bit bored.' But are you too worried about the can of worms that will be opened? Do you keep schtum and hope for the best? Or say it all and find a way through it? It's in your hands.

If you're Repowering it will inevitably influence your relationship. Do talk to your partner about it and be honest. Communication is always key. It's the foundation of every relationship. Often a partnership is in good shape, but you've just got out of the habit of talking. This can lead all of us to feel misunderstood or unheard, which, in turn, can breed resentment. Setting aside some undisturbed time to talk about your worries, hopes and dreams can be the key to Repowering a relationship. It really is amazing how much good a real, honest heart-to-heart can do.

Fern's Recipe for a
Repowered Relationship

- **It's just as important to listen as it is to talk – and when I say listen, I mean really *hear* what your partner has to say.** Try to actively listen, to repeat back what you've heard them say. Often, particularly if a conversation feels emotionally loaded, we can misinterpret what someone is saying. For example, they may say they'd like to spend more intimate time together and you might hear, 'You're boring in bed.'

- **Rather like rediscovering your vibrant teenage self, going back to the early days of a relationship can influence how it is today.** Think back and talk about what brought you together in the first place. Whatever it was, explore whether you'd like to revisit those activities together. Build on that. It's a good way to reconnect and create new memories together too.

- **Life happens so fast we don't often stop to tell our partners how grateful we are for all they do.** If you try to make it a habit to show your appreciation, they will most likely reciprocate and neither of you will feel as if the hard work you put in is going unnoticed. You can show your gratitude too with little surprises. They don't have to be grand gestures

– it's the thought that really counts. Leave them a note, pop a chocolate bar in their bag, plan a night out somewhere you know they'd really enjoy. We often do these things naturally at the start of a relationship but, as the years go on and you're weighed down by the responsibilities of adulthood, they can go out of the window.

- **While you're making plans together, take some time out for yourself, too.** It may sound odd to talk about spending time apart while we're looking at boosting our relationships but spending time apart is an important part of a healthy relationship. Pursue your own interests, spend time with your friends and you'll find it pays dividends for your relationship too. When you're feeling happy and fulfilled, you'll have a glow about you and will bring a lot more positive energy into your relationship.

- **When it comes to what people say they want in a new partner, a good sense of humour generally comes high up on the list.** So even if you've been together a long time, try to retain that sense of fun and laugh with your partner whenever you can. Laughing is marvellous for your health. There's science to back this up. It enhances your intake of oxygen-rich air, which stimulates your organs, increases endorphin levels, allays tension and long term it even boosts your immune system. And of course it enhances your mood. Plus, it's great for your relationship as it will strengthen your bond and makes life a bit more enjoyable.

- **Romance, too, is vital. It's often the glue that holds relationships together.** Rather like a fire, it will go out unless you keep it stoked. Keep flirting, holding hands, snuggling up on the sofa. It's these small things, rather than diamonds or five-star hotels, that keep the romance in a relationship alive. A girlfriend of mine once said: 'This man has allowed my ashes to go cold while I have been constantly tending his fire with extra logs and warmth to keep it going.' It's a telling image. We all need to feel we have our partner's attention.

- **It's important to remember no relationship is ever perfect.** The fact is that to be in any kind of long-term relationship means we need to be patient and forgiving with each other. All partnerships have ups and downs. Many relationships that seem strong from the outside have endured moments that almost ended them. Conflict arises in all partnerships and anyone who lives with someone else will know first-hand how infuriating the habits of others can be.

The trick, I think, is that when arguments happen (and the shouting has stopped), approach them with love and a desire to understand and compromise rather than to win.

- **There's also no point in hanging on to past misdemeanours, yours or theirs.** If you've chosen to go on with the relationship after a big blow-up, then try to move on as gracefully as possible, whether you were the one in the wrong or not. If it's worth saving, then save it. If you're overcome with guilt at something you've done that your partner may not know about – for example, you had a brief fling with somebody 20 years ago – it's probably best not to bring it up. Sure, it might help you feel unburdened, but you'll definitely cause unnecessary hurt and all over something that happened decades ago and will not be repeated.

Long relationships are not something we really celebrate in the way we do new ones. All fairy tales end just at the point of marriage. We don't get to see Cinderella and Prince Charming, five, 10, 20 or 30 years into the relationship. We don't know how he feels about the fact she never throws away her contact lens cases and leaves them in a little heap by the sink. We don't know if she is driven to distraction by the way he chews his food. I think this is rather sad – I would love to know if they celebrated their 50th anniversary.

Many of us can't even look to our parents as role models for a long and happy marriage. I certainly can't as my parents' marriage was over before I was born.

My Auntie Elsie and Uncle Paul did have a lovely marriage though and I really enjoyed spending time with them when I was growing up. Uncle Paul was my mum's older brother and he was like a father to me. As skipper of a Lancaster bomber in the Second World War, he won the Distinguished Flying Medal for bringing his burning plane back to base without losing any of his crew. I have a photo of him outside Buckingham Palace where King George VI pinned the medal on him. He was a fantastic uncle. Auntie Elsie was a brilliant housewife and a good mum to their two boys.

Uncle Paul and Auntie Elsie got married just before the end of the war. She had been part of the Women's Royal Air Force. To my young eyes, there was never any problem between them. She relished cooking and they both enjoyed doing the garden, and she would be listing jobs for him to do all the time. Uncle Paul loved Christmas so their house was magical at that time of year. He would hang decorations from the ceiling, swinging between the lights and at the corners of the room. Everywhere was twinkly and tinselly.

I would often go and stay with them as a little girl and everything just felt right, as if all was well in the world. There was a solid routine to life in their house. Everything felt smooth. I don't remember anything being at all tense. They were just a wonderful couple. They took in my grandmother when she was very ill and she stayed with them until she died. If it put any strain on their relationship, I never saw it; they only ever showed a united front. There was nothing showy about Auntie Elsie and Uncle Paul's relationship, but it had a solidity that felt comforting to me. What I took from their marriage is that a strong partnership and caring for and supporting each other are vital components of a healthy relationship.

One last point: if you think it would not be possible to have a full and frank discussion with your partner about your relationship, ask yourself why? Would you be met with aggression? Would you be put down? Would it all be spun around so that any problems are seen as being solely your fault?

If that is the case, maybe your relationship is coming to its close. Only you will know if it is over and, if so, you deserve a lot better.

Tips for Holding an Honest Heart-to-Heart with Your Partner

- Signal to your partner you need a serious conversation, but that there is nothing to fear.

- Explain that you need to resurrect some lost feelings inside yourself.

- Follow it by asking for five suggestions of things they would love to do.

- Brace yourself, then ask if there's anything they find irritating about you.

- Come up with a score out of ten for the current state of the relationship. And ask your partner to do the same.

- Assess the answers and ask yourself: are you best friends instead of lovers?

Chapter Nine

Love Me Tender, Love Me True

(Part 2)

We can't really talk about relationships without talking about sex. Surprisingly I am not a sex therapist but I can offer my own experience as a heterosexual woman. Mind you, having done ten years in daytime television, I often mistakenly think I am qualified to do a bit of everything.

So, here's a thing ... A recent study conducted by the International Academy of Sex Research revealed that gay men and women have more fulfilling sex (with gay men experiencing an orgasm 89 per cent of the time and gay women experiencing an orgasm 86 per cent of the time). Whereas when it comes to straight relationships, it was found that men orgasm an astonishing 96 per cent of the time and women only 65 per cent. This is called the orgasm gap and it's clearly a problem for straight women, but why is it happening?

Yes, why *is* it happening? As women, are we simply not spelling out exactly how we are able to orgasm successfully?

Or are men not too bothered about helping out? Gentlemen, may I remind you that 'ladies first' is a good place to start?

Interestingly, it was also found that those in homosexual relationships were 'more satisfied with their relationship, ask for what they want in bed and praise their partner for something they did in bed'. So, maybe there's a few lessons to be learned there.

Obviously, sex can be fantastic, exciting, thrilling and enjoyable and it usually is all of these things at the start of a relationship. Then life happens and you have to fit it in between doing the school run, the commute and the big Tesco shop. Real life takes its toll on a couple. At that stage it can feel a bit like, 'Oh no, not this again.' I always used to say that sex should be a hobby that you can both enjoy together. It doesn't cost anything. You don't need any special equipment. You can do it at home. You can go away and do it. How marvellous it would be when people ask, 'Are you doing anything this weekend?' to reply, 'Yes, we're having sex. We're awfully good at it.'

Talking to many female friends, it appears to me that the loving, the looking into each other's eyes, the feeling that you are the most desirable woman for your man starts to get lost. And so does the kissing. Kissing is a lovely and much undervalued part of foreplay in a long relationship.

Sex sometimes becomes less of a joint endeavour and more of a solo exercise for him. This is where women have to be honest; we are often our own worst enemies when it comes to speaking up about what we like and what is doing nothing for us. The thing that stops us is not wanting to hurt the feelings and the ego of our male partner.

There could also be an element of miscommunication going on. I recently read a theory that said women generally need to already feel close and connected with their partner before wanting to have sex, whereas for men, they find that sex *is* a way of connecting with their partner. It's this disconnect that can often leave couples misunderstanding each other's intentions. For example, if he instigates sex when you are not feeling particularly affectionate, you might feel like he just wants to get his rocks off, whereas he might actually just be wanting to love you. So the gap between you becomes wider. This is why communication is so important in a relationship to bridge this gap.

This is also where simple acts of kindness come into play. Talking to each affectionately, even if you're just doing the washing up together, can begin to start the magic. We all like to hear loving words from our partners. Little compliments. Asking how your day has been. Thoughtful actions like putting the bin out or reminding you that your favourite television programme is about to start.

I like tenderness and kindness. Growing up without a father, I think I missed out on the affection a father can give a daughter.

Last winter, when I had just had my shoulder fixed, I went for a walk in the village. It was around 5pm and it was cold and drizzly but I really needed some fresh air. I bumped into a neighbour whom I know a bit, and we exchanged pleasantries. As we stood chatting, the cold wind was going right down the collar of my coat and as my right hand was in a sling, I couldn't do the popper up. He saw me struggling and reached over and did it up for me. It was such a thoughtful thing to do and was done with a tenderness that I will never forget. That sort of thing really touches me.

If you and your partner don't speak the same love language or you didn't know about the concept, it's easy to put any sexual miscommunication down to a mismatch in libido when it might be more accurate to see it as a language issue. If you feel hugely loved when the bins are put out but your partner only gets this warm glow after physical touch, it's easy to see how things can get lost in translation. If you can communicate honestly and openly with each other about your love language then it's possible you'll end up having more sex while also never missing a bin collection. Sounds like a win-win to me.

While we're on the subject, lads, I must point out that a back massage is not foreplay. If you offer your partner one then do it in the spirit of generosity – not in the hope it will lead to anything more. Conversely, never, ever fake an orgasm. If you're spoofing, how does your partner know? Even if you've been pretending for years, stop right now.

You don't need to be harsh. You can say, 'That's great, but could you also try this?' The fact is, sex is only good if you both get something out of it. Putting your own happiness second – because you want him to be happy – isn't going to work in the long term.

Many people – particularly those who've been in the same relationship for decades – could do with a bit of Repowering in their sex lives. And now is a great time to get back into the swing of things in the bedroom. You probably have a bit more time. It is unlikely a three-year-old will burst in demanding a drink. However, as we get older, we might experience some physical issues around sex that lead to reluctance or difficulties. We all know the perimenopausal years and the menopause can cast a shadow on previously active sex lives and we also know that men can experience issues too as they age. Your doctor is there to help. Please don't feel embarrassed or shy going to talk to them. A good sex life is great for your physical and mental health, so if you're experiencing difficulties, it makes sense to ask for assistance.

One thing we don't often talk about when it comes to relationships is how both love and desire ebb and flow. Sometimes we completely adore our partners. At other times they drive us nuts. It's completely normal and nothing to worry about. What's important is to try to maintain a connection through good times and bad. It's not always easy, but it is worth the effort.

Small things can build up and become huge in your mind. Petty resentments are like little bricks. You must be careful not to build a wall with them. It's much better to talk everything through. To keep the lines of communication open, set aside time regularly to check in with each other. If you can tell your partner honestly how you feel about all areas of life, you might come away with a much-improved relationship or you might decide to go your separate ways.

If it's the latter it is, of course, hugely painful. Even when a relationship has run its course, it can be devastating when you both finally admit it's over. You do, though, have to think of yourself. If you've tried but it just isn't working, then really the best thing for both of you may be to just walk away.

Somebody I knew spent years putting up with a difficult relationship with her husband and one day her therapist said: 'Everyone's looking at your husband because he's splashing around in the pool, shouting, "Help me, help me!" while you're quietly drowning in the corner.' You have to ask yourself, are you willing to be the one who drowns and dies?

Some relationships are just plain unhealthy. If you have a partner who belittles you, is verbally or physically abusive, is controlling, isolates you, lies to you or does anything else that makes you uncomfortable then you have some hard thinking to do. There is help out there and, if you feel able to talk, your GP would be a good first port of call. Or, if you feel that's too big a step, then there are helplines such as the

one run by Women's Aid. It might just help to talk to someone and gently explore your options.

Other relationships end through no fault on either side.
It's sad but sometimes we just outgrow each other. The trick
here, I think, is to try to end it in a gentle and loving way.
Of course, it hurts and that's true even if you're the one
who is leaving. It's sad to see anything end, but sometimes
it is for the best.

You don't need to be bosom buddies with your ex, but
you can accept that you're weary warriors who have survived
together. And surviving peaceably together is way better for
the children than going to war.

Top Tips for Men for a Happy Wife

Feel free to rip out this page and give it to the man in your life!

- Make an effort to look your best. Women put a lot of effort into their appearance, so step up, have a shave and brush your teeth. You could even instigate a double bath or shower. That way you're both clean, nice and warm and it's a bit ooh la la!

- If you're going to buy flowers, make sure they're not from the garage. And if you're going to buy roses, you must either buy one or a dozen, nothing in between. If you want to buy more then they go up in multiples of dozens. Also, they don't always have to be red.

- When it comes to putting out the bins or emptying the dishwasher, do not tell your wife you've done it 'for her'. Big mistake!

- Doing the little things, such as producing a cup of tea or glass of wine, is always appreciated.

- Make her laugh; laughter goes a long way. It can even help when having small spats to introduce humour to defuse the situation. But do proceed with caution!

- Learn that a toilet doesn't clean itself.
- Show your appreciation for her and all the things she does for you. Make it a habit.

Chapter Ten

Mental Health Matters

*W*hen I came to Cornwall full time it made me realise that I'd been living my life at breakneck speed. Life down here happens at a much slower pace. When the holiday visitors arrive, they're still operating on city time, with life going at a million miles an hour in their heads. Cornwall runs at about two miles per hour. It's fascinating to see them slowly adjust. At first, visitors are impatient when they're held up in traffic but eventually, they just accept being stuck behind a tractor because the hold-up offers a chance to look at chalky clouds scudding across a vast blue sky, the gold of distant beaches and the stalky greens of hedgerows. It's part of a gradual transformation into the happy summer people they are bound to become, and their happiness is infectious. It's lovely seeing people enjoying themselves with their children, indulging in the simple pleasures of life.

Cornwall is the right place for it. Sitting by the sea is blissful. Watching the waves form then break, and form then break again is soothing. Sometimes – and this is a bit odd – I sit and look at the water and think about all the people that water has been through. John Lennon, Karl Marx, Elizabeth I, Taylor Swift. I mean, I think it's awesome.

I have struggled with depression since I was young – maybe even as a child – but never recognised it. I knew I wasn't as happy as I felt I should be. It was tricky. I was 18 and at drama school when depression was first diagnosed. The college doctor was very kind and opened my eyes to what this ennui was. I had recurring episodes through my twenties then after my boys were born I had postnatal depression, which was very challenging. I never seemed to be able to get ahead of myself. To be ready for the next feed or sleep. No matter how early I got up, I was always behind. So one night I hit on the idea of going to bed fully dressed so that I would definitely be ready for the morning. I continued to fool myself that I was all right, for a while, until I couldn't do it any more. The health visitor happened to be visiting for the boys and I was in tears. She asked what was wrong and I said: 'It's taken me three days to paint my toenails.' I was really sobbing, and she said: 'I think you need to see the doctor.' My mum was there and she made an appointment for that afternoon.

As soon as my mother left, I rang the doctor and cancelled the appointment. I was determined to keep up with the pretence that I was OK. Then, before I knew it, the doctor himself was on the doorstep. He was terrific and with his help I got a lot better. Remember how I mentioned earlier how it was good to accept help when it was offered? This was one of those times but I didn't realise it.

When I had Grace, my doctor kept an eagle eye on me, but things weren't great at home with my first husband, who had had to cope with me being unhappy in a way he couldn't possibly understand. He thought it was postnatal depression but I knew I was sad because our relationship was failing. My lovely GP made an appointment for me to see a psychiatrist who was known to be brilliant with postnatal depression. She was the tops. If I had PND she'd spot it. I had to wait a few weeks and my GP insisted I took my husband to the appointment.

At the hospital we waited outside in the corridor, and when the psychiatrist opened her consulting room door, she introduced herself by a different name. This was not the woman my GP had asked for, but a locum. Nevertheless, my husband and I trooped into her office and she began to ask all the usual questions about my childhood right up to the present day. A lot to get through. Finally, she sat back and said, 'When you're watching television, do you think they're speaking to you?'

Er, no.

'Do you hear voices?'

No.

'And when you're out and about, do you think people are staring at you and saying your name?'

Now this was at a time when I was presenting *Ready Steady Cook*, a show that was very popular and had many, many viewers. I was recognised everywhere I went.

So I said, 'Yes.'

'Ah.'

I saw something click in her eyes.

Instantly, I realised my mistake and said, 'No, because they do. I work in television!'

Now this woman was an academic, who would not have been watching afternoon television, especially not *Ready Steady Cook*!

Her response was meant kindly enough. 'You are psychotic. You need to be in hospital and on strong medication. We will phone you tomorrow.'

We got in the car and my poor shell-shocked husband didn't say a word. I was thinking, *Now he really thinks I am mad!*

The next day, the psychiatric department of our local hospital rang me to make an appointment for my admission. I said, 'That's very kind of you, but I'm fine.' She insisted: 'No, you're going to have to come in.' I said, 'No, I'm not,' and put the phone down. I rang my GP, who sighed deeply when I told him the story and told me he'd sort it. He must have contacted the hospital because I never heard from them again. And no, I did not have psychosis.

Later, I would tell this story as my warm-up joke for *Ready Steady Cook*. The audience loved it and by then I could laugh about it, which somehow made it all better.

When the doctor first suggested I start on antidepressants, after I had my boys, I had a lot of reservations, but he explained to me that they were simply 'a bridge across troubled water'. Life at the time was like a raging river and I had to get from one side to the other. They take effect slowly – it's not like taking a paracetamol for a headache – but after a couple of weeks I began to see the wood for the trees. They might not be suitable for everybody, I'm not necessarily endorsing them, but they really worked for me.

Depression takes any hostage it can. It doesn't discriminate, whether you're rich or poor, old or young, male or female. People think that if you have a great life, you shouldn't be depressed. But the truth is you never know when depression might hit you. It can strike at any time. So just be alert to how you're feeling now, particularly if you have experienced a big life change. The empty nest years, for example, can leave you feeling dissatisfied and dislocated, and that might creep up and grab you, taking you by surprise. (On the other hand, these years can be incredibly liberating!)

I have had a therapist for the past decade and we talk weekly. At the start of a therapy journey you may talk about your childhood experiences and then the challenges you have faced subsequently. Once that's done, you can begin to join up the dots from childhood to the present day to see how the child you once were has become the adult you are now. I run everything by her and have let go of a lot of old baggage I had been lugging about.

Therapy sessions take it out of you. I can't do anything for a couple of hours afterwards. I need to let it all just sink in. It will be working its way through your subconscious brain and doing an awful lot of good.

The waiting lists for NHS therapy are long and private therapy is expensive, but there are other options available, so it is well worth speaking to your GP if your mood is low. Subsidised therapy is available, as are self-help groups, and charities like Mind offer help as well.

If you are feeling depressed right now, I want you to know you are not alone. It is frightening when you are in the grip of it. You can have dark thoughts and they can be difficult to let go.

Everyone experiences depression differently. During my worst episode years ago, I felt the air was thick with tiny black particles, hanging in the air around me like a cloud of midges. I would wonder why others couldn't see this soupy mist. It was absolutely horrible but I survived and it's never happened since. In fact, I have been feeling well for several years now. Medication-free and grateful. But I'd like to offer some advice. I learned to recognise depression when it appeared on the horizon. Where previously I would have tried to run away from it and deny it, I discovered that if I stood still and let it pass through me, I would recover much more quickly. Weeks rather than months. I guess therapists would call it mindfully sitting and observing the feelings rather than pretending it isn't happening or blaming yourself for it and thinking, *I'm such a terrible person.* It's more: *OK, so I'm feeling this and this is happening …*

It is always a good idea to talk to people in your life about how you're feeling but you do have to choose wisely. Pick someone who is likely to be understanding. Blurting it all out to a friend who might not be sufficiently tuned in can be worse than not talking at all. That friend might say: 'Look at you, you've got everything you could possibly want. You have a lovely life in a lovely house and two holidays a year and you know you've got nothing to be sad about.' That's not the friend to choose because it will make you feel much worse. It's not their fault; they probably just don't understand because they haven't been there. But finding the right person to share your feelings with will make the burden feel a little lighter.

A GP may offer you some kind of antidepressant. It's worth considering this and talking through any concerns you might have with your doctor. People often worry that antidepressants will make them feel numb. Everybody's different, of course, but my experience is that they don't do that. Instead, they slowly made me feel more like myself again. It wasn't an instant cure, but I felt incrementally better after a few weeks. For me it was all about finding the right medication.

If you have a friend who is depressed, then don't feel you have to be a mental health expert to offer a little help. Start by making a cup of tea because, honestly, even boiling a kettle might feel like the most exhausting thing in the world to them. If you walk in and say, 'Right, sit down, I'm going to make you a cuppa,' that might make a huge difference to them. Then, if they want to talk, just sit and listen. Don't interrupt or add your personal experiences – they need to get everything out. And talking will make them feel a lot better.

As I have said before, my mum used to say, 'This too will pass.' And it will. As you start to come out of depression, you begin to feel a little more like yourself. If you're Repowering after an episode of depression, I urge you to take the process at a kind and slow pace. You will know when you are ready to attempt something small. Maybe you'll see a bag of knitting and think, *I'll finish that scarf,* or spot a half-used tin of emulsion in the shed and say, *I might paint that table today.* I have found it's all about doing only those things you can manage for just 10 minutes. So, take things slowly. My mum had an old doctor, a lovely man called Dr Patterson, who told her when she was rather low: 'Don't do anything you don't want to do.' I think that advice holds up.

Even when we're not suffering from clinical depression, many of us can be too black and white in our thinking, when many issues are firmly rooted in grey areas. There may not be a definitive answer, or a best result. Sometimes, it's the least worst outcome that we must accept, in order to go forward.

Catastrophising is another trap we can easily fall into and it can run rampant if it goes unchecked. When my boys came home after university, I tried very hard not to be one of those parents who keeps saying, 'When are you coming back tonight, who's driving and why don't you get a taxi instead?' They had had three years of being independent and I was suddenly acting as if they were 15 again. One night, I asked them to text me if they were staying over at a friend's house instead of coming home. No problem. Simple. The next morning, I opened my phone and saw there were no texts so I thought, *Good, they must be home in their beds.* But they weren't. Then I started thinking, *Where are they? Oh my God, they're probably upside down in a ditch! I'm going to have to call their dad, we're going to have to go to the hospital and identify the bodies!*

When they came home, I explained this to them (once I'd calmed down). They looked at me, astonished, and said, 'All that goes through your mind simply because we didn't send a text?' Since then they have been good at keeping me up to date with plans.

It is primarily but not exclusively the children I worry about. Sometimes the tiniest thing can blow out of all proportion. Here in Cornwall, I have a very tiny lawn and it currently needs to be raked up and started again. I don't want it seeded; I want it turfed. The gardeners were very keen to seed it. I was talking to Winnie and I said: 'They've asked me again if I'll have seed and I said no because the birds will come down and eat the seed and then our cats will eat the birds.'

Winnie said: 'Yeah, then a dog will come and eat the cats, and then a horse will come and eat the dog … It'll be just terrible. We'll have all these dead animals everywhere! And all because of the grass seeds.'

She was right to poke fun at me and, of course, it made me laugh. Laughing always helps puts things into perspective. It also made me realise the trick when you're catastrophising is to catch yourself as you're doing it. Once you start hearing yourself it can be quite amusing. Your brain says, *Everything is awful, everybody is terrible, everything is wrong, everybody hates me. Every, every, every …* You have to think, *Now hang on, that's not true, is it? I'm OK. Not everyone hates me. Things aren't so bad.* Maybe it's about trying to think of the worst-case scenario and then, when you can rationalise it, you'll see it's probably not the worst.

This kind of spinning out is more problematic when we are alone. Unfortunately, it's often true that when you finally pick up the phone and decide to talk to a friend, they'll be out. Dropped toast always lands butter-side down. When that does happen, I feel a relief that I don't have to put my burden on that person and it's a reminder that I can and will feel better tomorrow after a good night's sleep.

Speaking of sleep, as I get older, it's a constant battle to remember why I've come into a room, where my glasses are or what I'm meant to be doing that day. If I'm tired it's even worse. That's because sleep is vital for the memory. It's when we sleep that we cement new memories – a bit like uploading them to the cloud (whatever that is) – but sleep is also important for strengthening the neural connections that help us recall memories.

Relaxing is important. I can't stress this enough. I often just sit and stare into space. I wouldn't go as far as to say it's meditating, but sometimes, when the house is empty, I will just sit and think. Occasionally I go a bit further and try to let my mind go blank. A rest can just be five minutes with a cup of tea. Punctuate a day with those small things like a bit of lunch, a cup of tea, a piece of cake. Just take a little pause and enjoy it.

When I look back on the years my children were small, I was either at work, in the Co-op or at home with the children. Not the glamour you would expect. I look back and realise that I was longing for a moment when I could sit down and stare into space. Or just some time to read a book uninterrupted. Now is that time for me and I hope it is for you too. Now is our time to sit in a church or travel, eat good food, argue politics sensibly with another grown-up without worrying about the kids waking up.

Some people swear by naps as the key to keeping themselves on track. I am not a napper. That's not to say I don't fall asleep on the sofa in the afternoon, so I guess I do take the odd nap but never a planned one. Experts say napping is good for you. An optimum 20 minutes can help with cognitive function, give you an energy boost and make you feel more alert.

Sleep is crucial to wellbeing. I love to be in bed by 9pm, maybe even earlier. Some people enjoy fancy sleep routines, but mine is as ordinary as can be. I take my make-up off, I use a serum and some night cream, clean my teeth well, brush my hair, have a pee. And get into bed to watch some television or read a book. Then I have a think, get out of bed, have the last wee, go back to bed and turn the lights out. I'm usually asleep very quickly and I wake up very early. Five-ish …

Ensuring we get quality sleep is one of the most fundamental aspects of self-care. When we're sleeping well we tend to eat more healthily, feel less stressed and find it much easier to concentrate. While we're sleeping, our bodies repair and regenerate and getting the right amount of sleep helps strengthen the immune system. It's no coincidence that we tend to get colds or other viruses when we're tired and run down. Poor sleep has been linked to a number of chronic conditions including type 2 diabetes and obesity.

Not to get too technical, but sleep influences the way we process glucose and also our appetite-regulating hormones. This – and all the Mars Bars we consume when exhausted

– can lead to weight gain and the risk of obesity. Lack of shuteye has also been associated with high blood pressure, heart attacks and strokes.

I'm a huge fan of sleep. There are times when my battery is absolutely empty and I will say, 'I'm just going to go to bed.' It's generally when my mood is not so good. Then I might go to bed in the afternoon and disappear until the next morning. When I'm not feeling mentally strong, sleep is the best cure. I'm also very aware that I need to guard against tiredness as it can quickly lead to me feeling off kilter.

Being well rested means we will be able to concentrate better and be more productive. I'm sure you find, like I do, that solving problems is easier after a good night's sleep. Also, according to much research, you'll live longer if you're not sleep-deprived. Rather unfairly, apparently the effect for men is more powerful than for women. If they get the right number of hours in bed, they get a whole extra five years on the planet. Sadly, for us it's around two. (But we do live longer than the chaps overall.)

Stress is reduced if we sleep well as getting enough sleep allows our bodies to manage the stress hormone cortisol way better. All of this adds up to us being able to regulate our emotions more effectively. A lack of sleep can lead us to be moody, irritable and stressed out. A chronic lack of sleep is linked to mental health issues such as depression and anxiety.

When I don't get enough sleep, it leads to a real drop in mood and I can find myself getting grumpy. On that note, there is a saying that if you feel as if everyone hates you, you probably need to sleep. If you feel as if you hate everyone, you probably need to eat.

This isn't always the case, but sometimes if your mood is a little low it can be a good idea to try to think about anyone but yourself. Being aware of other people's struggles can put things into perspective a little and volunteering can be a powerful way of helping others and taking your mind off your own issues. Often this will give your self-esteem a boost as you'll feel a sense of achievement, belonging and satisfaction.

Whatever is going on in our world, we need to know that we are worthy of a happy and creative life. We need to get to the stage where we can put all that we have learned to good use and pass it on to others, where we can say, 'I've been there too, but it's all right.'

Finding Comfort in the Small Things

Don't underestimate the power of small comforts when you're having a really horrible day.

- My small comforts are varied and include big pants, *The Archers* and the BBC Sounds app, as well as time to finish a crossword in peace. Also, lashings of butter on crumpets!
- Revel in the real joy of small moments. I rejoice when I manage to conquer the self-checkout without asking for help! It doesn't happen very often but, when it does, it is like winning the lottery.
- The first cup of tea of the day.
- Walking around the garden and saying hello to the things I've planted as they emerge, year after year, having disappeared in the winter months.
- Managing to get all the cardboard flat and in the right bag to put out for recycling.
- Knowing that all three cats are somewhere in the house, safe and asleep. That makes me feel very good.
- A decent nightie is one that at a push you could wear to the beach and people wouldn't point and stare.
- Finally, clean bed sheets. If life is throwing you all kinds of sh*t, do yourself a favour and pop the bed linen in the wash. When you climb into bed that night, thank the earlier you who gifted this to you.

I don't think of this as anything as formal as practising gratitude, but I do think there are points in life where it helps if you can be thankful for literally the smallest of things. If you look around and think of five things you're grateful for, it can make all the difference …

Chapter Eleven

Families ...
We All
Have Them

*N*o matter how old your child is, being a mum leaves us in a constant state of anxiety or joy. Life goes so fast. One minute our babies are tiny and need all our attention, the next they're fully fledged, independent adults. So, job done – it's what we wanted, isn't it?

But then other feelings creep in. Suddenly, we're not the centre of their world any more and it stings. I would give anything to have one more day with my children when they were little and needed me. It's a lot to process when we're no longer the first stop in their lives and we start to ask ourselves difficult questions, such as, *Have I been a good enough mum?*

Motherhood brings with it so many lessons. We are not given a manual. When I had my twin boys, I was in a muddle, but I received some good advice which got me through. Such as keeping a diary as if I were at work, but instead of allocating meetings, I'd book in their needs instead. It helped me to see a structure in the day.

The second excellent piece of advice was to always put them down for a nap at the same time. It gave me moments in the day when I could I get the laundry out or maybe even sit down with a cup of tea. Beyond that, I had to work it out as I went along. The biggest lessons were that you never stop learning as a parent and that the demands of motherhood change with each stage of their lives.

Like all children, mine have had to face their own challenges, not least navigating their parents divorcing. Whilst not easy, divorce is not uncommon and it can help build resilience and understanding between parent and child if we communicate well. Answer all questions as truthfully as possible and without badmouthing your former partner. Their relationship with their other parent is not *your* relationship with their other parent! Blended families come with their own joys and challenges. Perhaps the hardest thing for children of any age is when a parent meets a new partner. I know that, aged nine, I found it difficult when my mother entered a new relationship. I adored her. She had been both mother and father to me and my sister. It's one of the reasons it was so hard when she met my stepfather. Another was that he was a difficult man. My stepfather was unused to daughters and now he had two. He was so in love with my mum that he became possessive. I felt as if I had lost her overnight. Suddenly there seemed no time for me to be alone with her any more.

My sister was old enough to have left home so it was just me and it was a lonely time. Silly rules came into force. I wasn't allowed to watch *Top the Pops*. I had to put money in a tin if I made a phone call on the home phone. If I spoke too much at dinner, especially when we had guests, he would shoot me a glance, and say, 'Empty vessels make most noise,' leaving me beetroot red and humiliated. He would introduce me to his friends as 'the youngest girl'. I had to knock on any door before I went into any room. I wasn't allowed to sit next to my mother on the sofa. Stupid, insidious, harmful stuff.

Sometimes I broke a rule I didn't even know was in force. One was that I had forgotten to kiss him goodbye when he dropped me at school. That evening he made a point of not picking me up from school, leaving me to wait for two hours. I waited by the shops, the agreed pick-up point, until it was dark and the shops were closing. I didn't know why I was in trouble, but I knew that this was some form of punishment. The nearest phone box was about five minutes away but I was frightened to walk down to it to ring home, in case he arrived and I wasn't waiting where I was supposed to be. When he finally picked me up, he said not a word to me. Not then and not for the next couple of weeks until I apologised. Just writing that down brings back the fear.

My dear mum was wonderful but was also careful not to upset him. However, there was one row, on her birthday, that ended in her walking out of the house and disappearing for hours. I watched her walk away down the front path wearing her black and white cheetah-print mac. She took nothing with her. My sister was home that weekend and we talked in whispers, wondering what had happened. My stepfather did not speak other than expecting my sister to cook the birthday lunch. It was chicken supreme and to this day I can never face eating it again.

He did give me £15 a month as my allowance but I had to pay for everything I needed, other than food. Clothes, shoes, underwear, haircut, toiletries. To be fair, it taught me the value of money and budgeting, and for that I am grateful. And, since I was buying my own things, I bought make-up and records, of which he disapproved, and went out with boyfriends, of which he also disapproved.

I am going to share something with you now that I have only told my children, as youngsters love to hear about the naughty things their parents once did. Here we go ... I was about 14 and every Sunday my job was to lay the dining-room table for lunch. I enjoyed this duty and enjoyed taking small nips of my stepfather's whisky from the sideboard (lunch in a slight haze was rather pleasant). But more than that, I got enormous pleasure out of watching my stepfather eating from cutlery I had spat on earlier.

A small but horrible act of defiance of which I am not proud, but ... it did make my children laugh.

In retrospect, I can see why my mum fell for him. He represented stability at a time when her existence was precarious. She'd recently lost her own mum and had to work hard to make ends meet. It was obvious to everyone that he adored her, so that must have given her a sense of security. But he was insecure in himself. For example, he didn't like that she was taller than him, so he didn't like her wearing high heels. Before they met, she wore glamorous stilettos and afterwards she started wearing flat shoes.

As my stepfather aged, he mellowed and, as I grew older, I could better understand him. When I was in my forties, he was diagnosed with Parkinson's disease, and then prostate cancer, so his personal power began to ebb. My mum became a carer for him until she was exhausted and could do no more. My sister rang saying he needed to go into a home. They had found a place for him, but she asked if I would fund it. I said that of course I would.

I was the last person in the family to be with him before he died. He was in bed and wasn't breathing very well. The nurse had to come to clear his chest by putting a tube down his throat. She asked if I wanted to leave the room, but I said, 'No, I'll help.' We changed his pyjamas and got him comfortable. He died just a few hours later. It felt good to have helped him. It wasn't exactly a reconciliation, but it did close that chapter of my life.

I know that many blended families work brilliantly but there are trip hazards galore. Incoming step-parents have to tread carefully, while children struggle to maintain loyalty to both their mother and father. We must remember that children often don't have the language or the experience to express their feelings, so it is up to the adults to have patience and understanding when a child reacts badly.

I have been lucky that both my husbands have been loving fathers to our children and we have all muddled through. I wish that things had turned out differently and that my children didn't have to see their parents get divorced, but all I can do is apologise, be there for them and try to understand how they're feeling.

My children are incredible. I don't talk too much about them because I value their privacy. They're adults with their own stories to tell, but I'm tremendously proud of them and think, *Wow, you're incredible and you don't need me, so something is good. You are so independent.* And yet, if I'm being honest with myself, there's still a bit of me that just wants them to say, 'Mum, can you help?'

Repowering becomes essential when the nest is finally empty. It feels so odd to have no children at home. A quiet descends that is quite disconcerting, particularly if you have had several children. Many women suffer when the last of their children leaves home. Empty nest syndrome is real and can be brutal. The house can feel eerily quiet and strangely bigger without their clutter. Not having to think about meals and refilling the fridge can feel odd, too. It takes a while to get into the routine of shopping and cooking for just one or two.

This is your opportunity to start redefining your role and how you view yourself, and then you can start Repowering. It's useful at this stage to remember we are in charge of our own lives. Only we can Repower. Nobody can make us do it and nobody can stop us. It's like quitting smoking. You have to want to do it, otherwise you're not going to succeed.

If we try to turn our children into people who exist only to make us happy, whose choices can make us miserable, then we're doomed to failure. Celebrate the path they're taking, show interest in it but don't pester for information. I fall into the trap of messaging my children too often and with lots of questions. I appreciate that can feel like I'm a mum who is trying to be too present and I need to back off a bit.

I'm aware that I need to stop offering help and advice when it hasn't been sought. The small people who once told you their every thought now leave you desperate to know what's going on in their lives. Don't push them. If they do sit down and open up to you, try not to interrupt. I struggle with this because I feel I have to say something affirming or sensible. I must resist. It's hard because it's wonderful and scary to see that little person who used to sit on your hip, who would come in at two in the morning saying, 'I can't sleep,' all grown up. It makes me a little teary now because they're so wonderful. If they do ask for advice, make a point of listening properly before you try to guide them and appreciate that your own life experience isn't always a useful comparison to what they're going through.

Of course, empty nests aren't necessarily final outcomes and often children seem like they are on elastic. Winnie got a summer job working at a beach café, with the opportunity to rent a house with a couple of friends. Off she went and it was the first time in 29 years that I had been on my own, with no children at all.

I missed her horribly, but I quickly began to love the tranquillity and the tidiness. And she'd be back in six months, so I knew the unaccustomed silence was a temporary one. It was good for both of us to test the water. She was glad to come home again to get the laundry done in a nice warm house with food in the fridge, where no one would forget to buy the milk. She and I appreciated each other more, I think, when she got back.

I was thrilled when she returned. She's my 'man about the house'. She's got the biggest and best tool kit of anyone in the whole village and some of the guys ask to borrow her tools. She's very practical. She can do anything. She's earning money in construction at the moment. She's literally on a site, helping to erect a building. Two builders have taken her under their wing and she is doing really well. When I see her up on the roof with her nail gun, it makes me proud.

Even when she was little, she could make anything. She's also very good at sewing, even without a pattern.

It might not seem like an easy thing for a mother and adult daughter to live together but we're having a great time. Like all of us, both she and I have bright moods and our dark moments. When that dreary veil descends, we take ourselves off to be alone. It doesn't threaten our domestic harmony. Winnie often wants to watch programmes I don't like. So, she'll watch on her iPad with her cans on her ears and I'll watch TV with the subtitles on. Sitting next to each other on the sofa, or at least in the same room, it's one of the small joys of the end of the day.

Of course, children can miss their parents, too. Grace went off to Norway for a year on the EU Erasmus programme when she was at university and had an incredible time. But I remember when we were speaking on the phone once, her suddenly saying, 'Oh, I miss you, Mum.' Which was very well received.

If you're no longer with your child's other parent, it's important that your children, of whatever age, spend time with them without you creating a big drama or making your son or daughter feel guilty. This is also the case when your ex meets a new partner and your child will then be spending time with a different family. In-law envy is surprisingly common.

You will always be their mum. But it's your choice as to what sort of mum you're going to be. The choice is to either be the easy, accepting, loving mum or the mum whom no one wants to invite for tea or Christmas. High days and holidays can also take some processing for the single parent and not having the children home for those dates takes a bit of getting used to. Emotional blackmail (of which we are all capable) will not serve you well.

That's when Repowering can be such a useful tool. It can help you let go. It incorporates that Buddhist thing: you love people but can't expect them to feed your happiness. In Buddhism, you are taught not to grasp or cling to something external for your wellbeing. I must not, cannot, should not – in fact none of us should – rely on someone else to make me happy because that is never going to happen. We are all responsible for our own happiness.

This year, it turned out that all my children spent Christmas elsewhere. It required a bit of pre-planning to get my head in the right space so I could be sure I wasn't going to be accosted by any unwanted negative feelings. But I had decided there was no way I was going to feel sorry for myself.

I woke up early on Christmas morning and had a chat with the cats. I gave them all a tickle, said happy Christmas and made their breakfast, before going for a run. When I got back, I took some time getting myself bathed, dressed and made up for church. After I came downstairs, I opened my presents, which was hugely cheering as there were some lovely ones. I was rather spoiled as there were around ten parcels. Wonderful things from the children and Two Cups and Boo, and other friends.

Then I collected myself up and went to church, which was joyful. The year before, the church had been absolutely jam-packed. So much so they had to put out folding chairs in the aisles. Communion took an age as there were so many queuing for wine and wafers. This year it wasn't as packed, but it was full of all the best people. No one was made to feel like a stranger. There were holidaymakers there as well – who are always welcome – but it always feels like a proper congregation. That morning it was the very best place for me to be. It felt both Christmassy and peaceful.

After church I went for a walk on the beach. It was almost empty, but I did bump into a few people I knew. Each of them invited me to join them at home: 'You must come and have lunch,' or 'I can't bear for you to be on your own.' It was great that I could honestly say I was fine and was looking forward to the day alone. The tide was out, making the beach huge, so I walked all the way down to the water and back before making my way home.

As a treat, I made myself my favourite lunch – a lamb chop with new potatoes, peas and gravy – and watched television with the cats around me. Then I sat and did some writing. At various stages throughout the day the children rang, bringing extra joy.

In the end – although some people might have been a bit nervous about the prospect of spending the day alone – it was really relaxed. It genuinely was a great day. It worked so well, I think, because I planned what I wanted to do, so my brain was prepared. And it paid off. The next day, Grace came for lunch with her boyfriend and their two dogs, which gave me that Christmassy feeling, just 24 hours later. I am proud of my 'grand-dogs'. They are adorable. One day I hope to have human grandchildren but I fight off the urge to nag my children about this. I don't want them to feel as if they're under any pressure. But I was ready for them yesterday!

A word on grandparenting. I see so many grannies offering to help out a little, when the babies are tiny, and finding themselves still on the school run 15 years later. So, if I ever find myself as a grandparent, I do not want to fall into the trap of becoming a 'nanny granny'. I will draw the lines early and agree the terms. This may sound selfish but remember that word 'self-ist' we touched on earlier; we also need to think about our own needs. We are at a stage in life where we have loosened our ties to home and family and wish to enjoy the life we have left. Travelling without worry or guilt is the thing I most look forward to. This does not rule out looking after our beloved grandchildren, but we should not be enslaved to them (or their parents!). I say all this now, but who knows what will happen in the future.

As they grow into adulthood, you might find your children are not following the path you wanted or expected for them. They can't all grow up to be doctors, solicitors or the prime minister. Drop your preconceived ideas. Listen to them and listen some more. As long as they are happy, that's all that's important. Stop thinking of them as children. They're adults. They're independent. They are their own people handling their lives the way they want. For me, it helps to remember how independent I was at their age and to remember how very much the world has changed since I was young.

Even as a child I was independent. There was an age gap between me and my sister. When she left home aged about 17, I was eight. I have always enjoyed my own company and sitting quietly reading a book. At my small pre-prep school I won the reading cup three years in a row. Because I got that hat-trick, I was given a small replica of the actual cup to keep. I still have it. It is engraved with my name, Fifi Britton, and the year, 1965. The other prize was a book token so I went off to WHSmith in Gerrards Cross and bought a book called *A Treasury of Fairy Tales*, published by Collins. It is beautifully illustrated and has all the best fairy tales in it, from Snow White via Puss in Boots to The Frog Prince. There is a piece of typed paper glued to the blank inside page which reads:

LITTLE TURRET SCHOOL

Presented to Fifi Britton for general
good work throughout the year.

Elsie Bird [the signature of our head mistress]
July 1965

I am SO proud of that cup and book! By the way, Fifi was my nickname. It was so widely used that I didn't realise my real name was Fern for a long time.

Apart from reading, I also loved the freedom of cycling. I think that a bike must be one of the greatest things made by man. It's up there with the discovery of fire and of course the invention of the wheel (somewhat essential to bikes). When I wasn't exploring the lanes of the village, I was in the garden. We had a rainwater butt and I loved the sound of it. If I swished the water with a lump of wood I could pretend I was on a boat on the river, rowing along. The reading and the solitude all fed my imagination and have brought me to where I am today.

Times have changed since I was a child. I grew up on the war stories and bravery of my mum, uncle and aunt. You'll remember my uncle was a Lancaster bomber pilot but did I tell you my mum was a sergeant in the Auxiliary Territorial Service, the women's branch of the British Army? She was a predictor on the heavy ack-ack guns that shot down enemy aircraft. As a little girl I was, and still am, so proud of her and her stories, that when she would ask me, 'Who won the war, Fifi?', I'd say, 'You did, Mummy.' She loved it.

The world seemed a happier, more flourishing place when I was young. If you didn't want to go on to A-levels there was banking, nursing, the RAF or a host of other well-paid jobs from which to choose. Then you could set yourself up in a rented place while you saved for a deposit on a house. Nothing seemed out of reach. Aged 23, I managed to buy my first home, a tiny two-up, two-down Cornish cottage for £15,000 and I got a 100 per cent mortgage. How mad does that sound now? Today, kids can't even dream of buying a house. When you look at the difference in salaries compared to house prices, it's never going to match up.

Young people today are navigating a very different world to the one we grew up in. They've lived through so much already with the Covid-19 pandemic, the war in Ukraine and the Middle East, and, of course, the existential threat to the planet posed by climate change. Accidentally, unknowingly, unwittingly, we've deprived them of a certain future. It's easy for them to ask why they should care about anything as the whole thing feels as if it's going to implode any minute and they might not survive. Winnie and a few of her friends talk this way a lot. It's horrible to hear but also completely under-standable. This generation may never own their own home. Or pay off their university debt. They may decide to never marry or have children. They may decide to live halfway across the world. Remember, though, that they are still the people we love and admire. We must never lose sight of that.

There are other aspects of modern living that might seem outside our experience. Maybe their sexual orientation or gender identity confuses or panics you. But should your child approach you about their experience of sexuality or gender, it's important to listen to them and really *hear* what they're saying. If they say, 'I think I'm bisexual or asexual or pan-sexual,' or they say, 'I'm a woman in a man's body,' or 'I'm a man in a woman's body,' just listen. Let them know they have all the time they need to work themselves out. There is no rush. Read up about these things and be supportive and understanding.

The new understanding of pronouns can also be a bit muddling. If someone lets you know their preferred pronouns, please don't roll your eyes. There are two reasons for this:

1. It's the way this person wants to identify themselves. We must respect that.
2. To do so makes you look outdated. And that is NOT what we Repowerers are!

We all like to have our needs considered. To have a family, security, a roof over our heads, enough food to eat. To have friends and the respect of others. That's all we want. That's it. That's the recipe for being human. You can make somebody's life sheer hell by tearing them apart, pulling them down and destroying their confidence if you want to, but you can be sure it's going to come back and bite you on the bum. It's impossible to be human and not to struggle and we all need to be a bit more aware of that. We don't know everything that's going on in each other's lives and a bit of kindness goes a long way.

Often just as we're dealing with our children growing up and leaving home, our parents get to the age where they need to lean on us a bit more. Yup, you find yourself bang in the middle of tricky children who worry you more than ever and elderly parents who, well, worry you more than ever. What shall we do with Granny? Watching our parents age is a bittersweet experience. On one hand, we feel grateful for the time we've had with them. On the other, there's a sorrow in seeing them struggle with the challenges ageing brings. It's perfectly normal to feel sad, helpless and even a bit frustrated. We shouldn't feel guilty if we struggle with our emotions around this. It's hugely challenging.

If your ageing parent or parents are in good cognitive health, it's important to talk to them now about finances and care. Have they written their will and is it up to date? Without one, they will have unthinkingly left you in a quagmire of legalities. Having a will means their wishes will be clearly stated and will save potential conflict. (Remember, where there's a will, there is a family!) Would they accept you taking on the role of lasting power of attorney? There are two types: one for health and welfare and the other covering property and financial affairs. Believe me, it makes sense to get one for both. It will save you a lot of heartache in the future and will allow you and them to make decisions in accordance with their wishes. Talk to them about their preferences when it comes to any care needs they may have. Discuss how you can balance your own life with helping them and be honest about how much time you can commit. Juggling a career and caring for parents is obviously utterly exhausting, mentally, physically and financially. Don't try to do everything yourself. Reach out to siblings, if that's possible, to share the load. If you're an only child, look into professional support.

Care homes are expensive and it's important to find one that suits your parents' needs. They can be amazing places if you have one that is a good fit. My father was in a nursing home for actors and it was excellent. There were old scripts all over the place. My father often had one in his hand. He was 95 and suffering with dementia, but loved the idea that he had a job to do. I had great conversations with him about his job. He'd tell me, 'You know, I'm in a marvellous play – director's wonderful, absolutely wonderful. I'm not sure about rehearsals. I'm not sure what we're doing in rehearsals.'

The leading lady, of course, was always in love with him. It was all a fabulous fantasy. I used to take in alcohol-free beer and my father and his resident brethren would drink it and say, 'Well, this is awfully good – jolly good stuff this.' I had checked beforehand that it wasn't going to interfere with any of their medicines and they seemed to enjoy it.

When dealing with anyone with dementia, it is best to go along with what they are saying. If they ask, 'Where's your mother?' and she is dead, it's better to say, 'She's just popped out,' or 'She's on holiday.' My father often asked me how my mother was or asked after his second wife, my brother's mother, who had also died. I would just say to him, 'They've gone on holiday – together.' 'Really? And are they happy?' 'Yes, they're having a wonderful time.' 'Well, isn't that marvellous.' What is the point of saying, 'She's dead'? It only leads to more grieving and confusion.

Towards the end of my father's life, my sister and brother were there a lot and I'd been visiting frequently too, but was now living in Cornwall so I had said my goodbyes a little while before. It was very close to Christmas when we got the call from his partner, Jane, and she simply said, 'He's gone.' It was OK. It was peaceful.

As children all we can do is offer our parents the care we would like to receive when we get to that sort of age. Of course, not all of us have had happy childhoods or indeed a close relationship with our parents and I recognise that it can be much harder to care for elderly parents in those circumstances. I have huge sympathy and compassion for you if you're in this position. Make sure you grab a few minutes for yourself whenever you can. Even if it's just to sit quietly with a cup of tea or to have a warm bath. It's hugely important to take care of yourself.

Not all parents will suffer from ill health and I know many people well into their later years who are having an absolute ball. If you have a parent like this, it's a double-edged sword. It's marvellous that they're still having a great time, but you don't stop worrying about them. Personally, I'm looking forward to a time when I can be just like my stepmother, who flies like a swallow off to the sun, whenever she can.

Tips on Parenting

- Don't be too hard on yourself. We parents don't always get it right but if there are things you regret about your parenting style, just apologise whole-heartedly. Fractured relationships can be mended.

- Never employ emotional blackmail! It's tempting and easier said than done to resist, but guilt-tripping your child into anything will push you further apart.

- What was your relationship like with your own parents? Were they too pushy? Or always wanting something? Did you dread the phone calls? That's maybe how your children are feeling about you! Ease up and ease into your new role as a laid-back, kind, helpful (when asked), proud parent.

- And remember: all children want parental approval. Yours will be no different.

Chapter Twelve

Making It Work

A career change is great at making us feel dynamic again and a good way to examine what really makes us tick. Think back to moments when you felt on top of the world at work. What are you good at? What do you love? Pinpointing these things can help steer you onto new opportunities.

When I was working on *This Morning*, my life became so fast-paced that I didn't have a moment to register all the amazing things I got to do. I'd go home and someone would ask what was on the show that day, and I'd reply, 'Can't remember.' My brain literally couldn't compute what I'd done just a few hours previously. But now I have time to reflect on bits I had forgotten. Very often when a famous name pops up in the papers or on television, I can't help but say, 'Oh I interviewed them.' It's happened so often now that the girls joke back, 'We're putting that on your gravestone, Mother.'

Of course, Repowering doesn't have to involve a change of job like it did for me. Perhaps you might be suffering from *quiet quitting*, which is when you mentally check out while still being physically there at your desk. Doing the minimum required of you and avoiding anything extra. It usually happens when someone feels stressed and burned out, overwhelmed and unappreciated. If that's you, be honest with yourself: is that really the way you want to live? It's time to Repower and make a plan. We all have times when we simply can't give everything we have to work. We're human, after all. And we can change things.

It's good to look back over our careers and pick out the moments, the assignments, the projects, the periods of real creativity or invention that fired us up. Maybe your job involved dealing with people and you can pinpoint whose life you improved or where you excelled.

At the start of my career, I spent 13 years in newsrooms, which most people don't know. I learned how to be a journalist on the job. I was at BBC Plymouth in 1982, when the Falklands War began, and, for my generation, this was a first. We hadn't experienced a country's call to arms and I remember the buzz of activity in the newsroom. The maps came out, as no one was quite sure where the Falklands were or why it would take the Task Force six weeks to get there. Most of us were sure they were just off the Orkneys! As we were based in a naval city, we were on high alert, watching the news unfold. We watched as Royal Navy ships left Devonport for the long voyage to the other side of the world.

On the morning of 5 April 1982, the fighting unit 42 Commando from the Royal Marines left Plymouth to join their ship in Southampton. The Plymouth Registrar's office opened at 7am for the men to marry their sweethearts. I acted as a witness for one of the couples. Their wedding had been hastily arranged and there were many tears as they left the Registrar's office as man and wife, with no time for consummation. I travelled with them as they went straight to the parade ground. It was an incredible sight. Many, many men, in battle dress, highly trained, ready to fight and ready to lose their lives. Their Commander-in-Chief stood on a dais in the centre of the parade ground and delivered a moving speech. Inspiring and honest. He knew there were men around him who would not return. His final words were: 'Quick march – the South Atlantic.' Cutting through an atmosphere laden with dour expectation, it brought tears to my eyes and I will never forget that day. All the servicemen then said goodbye to their wives and girlfriends, including the couple whose wedding I'd just witnessed, and boarded several coaches to take them to Southampton and the aircraft carrier HMS *Hermes*.

As well as looking to the past and what we've witnessed previously in our working life, we should also look for inspiration in the present. Look out for courses and workshops that inspire you and see if taster sessions are available. Even if you decide it's not for you, you'll probably meet some interesting people and it might ignite a passion for a new hobby – and that might lead to a business opportunity.

Who wouldn't want to turn a hobby into a job? For example, I'd love to work in a gardening centre or in a library, or train as a masseuse. It's great to get paid for a passion. Side hustles offer a path to meet new people and get involved with the community. Although my career has been dominated by television and writing, I've had other ideas along the way.

There was a time after I left *This Morning* when I decided to train as an acupuncturist and learn Chinese medicine. I went off to a small college in north London to secure a place on the relevant course and I bought all the books, but it went out of business so that didn't happen. It was a shame as I thought I'd be good at it. After that I was going to retrain as a midwife. I'd thought I was too old but, when I asked at the hospital, it turned out I wasn't. Then life took over so that didn't happen either.

Every programme I have worked on, from news and current affairs through to cooking, gardening and interviewing film stars, means that I have a smattering of knowledge across all subjects, but I recognise I am a Jack of all trades … master of none.

When I started on TV, I was seen as a bit of an action girl! I once did a piece to illustrate how the RNLI air-sea rescue operations work. I was taken out in a small boat off the beach at Looe and dropped into the sea. So, there I was, bobbing about in the water like a cork, smiling and rather enjoying myself. Then I heard the helicopter and thought, *Oh good, here it comes.* But as it got closer, it was very noisy and the downdraft from the rotor blades whipped up the sea so much that I genuinely thought I was drowning!

Out of the side of the helicopter appeared a man on a wire who looked at me intently while giving me the thumbs up. He snapped a harness on me and wrapped me inside his arms and legs, then looked up and gave the helicopter above the signal. As the winchman started to wind us in, I felt so secure and out of danger. It was like a movie ending. I sort of fell in love with him: my rescuer, a knight in a shining wetsuit.

That was one of my most exciting adventures, and the point I'm making is that it is entirely in my nature to say yes first and worry about the consequences later. Don't give me a challenge because I'll just do it. My middle names are Gung and Ho! I've learned in life that it's never worth going for the safer option. Safety can smother creativity. The old adage, find a job you love and you'll never work a day in your life again, is true. So, I have always tried to choose a job I knew I'd love. And if I made a mistake in the process, that was fine; the sky didn't fall in. I could look around for something else.

I'm most proud of a series of films I did for *This Morning* in 2007 where I visited the British troops stationed in Basra, Iraq. At the time we were hearing that their equipment was substandard compared to the Americans'. I wanted to show the servicemen and -women's worried families who were left back home how their loved ones were living and working.

We took off from Brize Norton in a plane filled with soldiers; some were only 17 and this was their first deployment. I couldn't imagine how their parents must be feeling. To their credit, they were all positive, emphasising how well trained they were, but also acknowledging some nerves. We flew around Europe, dropping off and picking up troops, until we finally got to the Middle East and landed in Kuwait. The film crew and I got out of the plane in the middle of the night, then we were put in a Land Rover and taken to a perimeter fence where we were left to wait in the dark and eerie silence of the desert. There was a point when I wondered if we were doing the right thing! But eventually another Land Rover appeared and we were taken to our hotel and told to stay in our rooms for 24 hours. Nobody knew we were in the country.

Then, at three o'clock the next morning, we did the reverse; we were collected and dropped at the perimeter fence where another Land Rover came to collect us and drive us to a small hut near the air strip. We waited for a few hours and then a Hercules transport plane arrived and we hastily boarded. As we flew over the border into Iraq, I was invited into the cockpit and saw the oil fires on the horizon. The pilot told me that we now had to turn off all the lights illuminating the aircraft, to make us less visible to the tracer fire coming towards us. He also employed 'tactical manoeuvring' where the plane dips from side to side and noses up and down to literally dodge the bullets. I have often been asked if I was scared but I wasn't. I had absolute faith in the pilot and the aircraft.

Eventually we landed and we all ran off the back of the plane, me wearing my helmet and flak jacket with the words PRESS printed on the front, so that, in any dangerous situation, we would be immediately recognised as civilians. When I looked back, the plane was already heading for take-off. It would have been a sitting duck if it had waited a moment longer.

The Basra base was known as the Contingency Operating Base (COB) and I was put in what was described as 'VIP accommodation' – a steel shipping container with a single bed and a small shower. The wind had brought in a lot of sand so it was a bit gritty in there and the shower had a notice on the wall saying no shower could be longer than two minutes, as water was precious. That first night, the siren went off and I did what I had been told to do in a safety briefing. 'Keep your flak jacket and helmet on the floor by the bed so you can get straight into them. Lie on the floor with your mouth open and your hands cupped over your ears. The space under your fingers will help prevent your eardrums being blown. Keep your elbows close against your ribs to shield your core from shrapnel.'

I heard the incoming rocket fire whistle towards the camp before a decided *CRUMP* as the rocket made impact. I wasn't frightened at all; I was too busy concentrating on what I'd been told to do. When the all-clear sounded, I dusted myself down and went back to bed. The next day, my director, Verina, and I were out filming when a siren went off again. We immediately hit the deck and adopted the position. As we heard rockets whistling by to our right, a man in civilian clothes appeared and stepped over us. Calmly, he remarked, 'It's all happening a long way away. Nothing to worry about.' Verina and I exchanged a look of disbelief and stayed where we were on the ground. We didn't get up until the all-clear sounded. When I got home and told the children about that, Grace said, 'You never hear the blast that kills you.' I don't know how she knew that, but this was later confirmed to me by an ex-serviceman.

The whole assignment was amazing. We went on helicopter gunships and tanks. We talked to doctors, the chaplain and other men and women there, learning what all their jobs entailed. They were dedicated, hard-working and many of them were so young. It was humbling. I was only there for three nights, and I wouldn't have missed a second of it. My mum was desperate to hear all about it when I got home.

Of course, not all my assignments have been so gritty and dangerous. Certainly, over the years, I've been lucky enough to have encountered a bit of glitz and glamour in my line of work, too.

Like everyone else, I've always had heroes and, thanks to my job, I've met some of them. Singer Dionne Warwick appeared on *Fern Britton Meets ...* in 2012 and we talked about her fight against racial segregation and her grief following the death of her cousin, Whitney Houston. Despite her celebrity status, she arrived without an entourage and wearing a luxurious fur coat. It was, after all, December. When I asked if I could try it on, she agreed, and then I cheekily asked her, 'Can I have it when you're dead?' Quick as a flash, and laughing, she replied, 'You'll be dead before I am.'

In 2016, I met Bette Midler! My brother was playing Henry IV for the Royal Shakespeare Company in Brooklyn, USA, and Bette Midler had come to watch the show. For 40 years I've been a huge fan of hers. I love all her work. I'm not embarrassed to admit that I know most of the lyrics to *Live at Last*, her first live album, released in 1977, and it's a double one to boot! Am I fan-girling too much?

So back to that night in Brooklyn and there she was, sitting a couple of seats away from me with her daughter. She was dressed quietly and elegantly, hair neat, specs on, wearing a well-tailored pair of trousers and a lovely jacket. She was sharing a bag of M&Ms with her daughter. SO NORMAL!

After the show she had made it known that she wanted to go backstage to meet the cast. I was also going backstage to see my brother and so we went as a little party, the three of us. She was lovely and very easy to chat with as we climbed the stairs to the dressing room. I told her that my brother was the lead and she was impressed because he was so very good. She asked me what I did and I sort of mumbled something about television and then, at the top of the stairs to greet us, was my brother, waiting outside his dressing room. I introduced him to Bette and her daughter. I could see his eyes light up and we both tried our best to keep it together. She then asked: 'Hey, should we have a picture?' Yes, please! I mean, here's this immensely talented STAR asking if we'd like a picture! And there she was, standing between me and my brother with her daughter taking the shot.

She's one of only three women I've met who have a special shimmer about them (Dolly Parton and Princess Diana were the other two). Some kind of fairy dust that even when they've left the room is still shimmering in the air. I wish we could bottle some of that fairy dust for all women to believe in our own power.

It's great to see other women doing well and there's something very powerful about women supporting each other in the workplace. Female friendship – or even just passing interactions – can have a huge impact on us. A few years ago, I was doing a show called *Time Crashers* and worked with Kirstie Alley from the US cult series *Cheers*. We were travelling around all over the place on location and were put up in little cottages.

So, she and I being the, ahem, old ones, we were always up with the lark while everyone else was asleep. She loved drinking tea and was amazed that I would make it every morning with a teapot and a tea cosy. I'd take it out to the garden on a tray for her while she was having a cigarette. She was a fabulous woman. She would tint her eyebrows over the kitchen table in those rented cottages and looking into a mirror and would say to herself, 'Oh, hello lovely lady. You're very beautiful.' I loved that. Most of us look in the mirror and see only our flaws. She always called me Fernando. 'Fernando, Fernando, come here!' I absolutely adored her.

The director on the show was called Simon, and he was very handsome. Now, Kirstie and I enjoyed showing off our bendy yoga skills to each other when we had time to exercise, and one morning she asked me if I'd ever seen the 'director pose'. No, I hadn't. 'Let me demonstrate for you, Fernando.' She got down on all fours, her face maybe four inches off the floor, and then said, in her husky, unmistakeable voice, 'Oh, *hello* Simon.' I cried laughing.

I have worked with some fantastic women over the years. Daytime television attracts a lot of highly skilled women, both in front of and behind the cameras. It makes the workplace so much more fun and we all understand the pitfalls and internal politics we face. Ageism against women is not quite as blatant as it was in the 1980s when, as women, we just had to tolerate behaviour that would be nipped in the bud nowadays. But it still exists, and between our early fifties and retirement we may feel passed over and less relevant. Many studies show that both women and men come up against age discrimination in the workplace. Women, though, tend to experience it earlier – at 45 – compared to 55 for men. Certainly, there are still more older men on screen compared to women.

Being a working mum is not easy. The work-life balance is tricky and after I had children it did become hard. But I was very lucky in that I had three part-time nannies: my mum, Super Sue and Karen (aka Camel). Between them the workload was shared so that no one was exhausted. I would be home by the time the children came back from school, so breakfast was the only part of the day I missed with them. I never wanted the children to think work was more important to me than they were. On one occasion, I was told live on air via my earpiece that Grace was being taken to hospital. As we were coming up to a commercial break, I asked if I could leave and miss the rest of the programme. The answer was a resounding yes and I ran straight out of the studio. But to be honest, even if they'd said no, I would have gone! Poor Grace had cellulitis under her eye and needed intravenous antibiotics. I stayed by her side for the next two nights.

Seeing my children grow up was wonderful and the love that I have for them is fierce, but it doesn't help anyone if we don't acknowledge the fact that for women it is harder to balance a career with small children.

These days I look back and recognise how lucky I was to have such a lovely family and a job I loved. I urge you to take a minute and look back at everything you've done ... so far. Appreciate it and be proud of all you have achieved and all that is still to come.

Repowering is helping me pull up the positives. Even with all the bear traps that I've fallen headlong into, my life has been incredible. I've been given gift after gift after gift and I'm now determined to appreciate them all. Most of us have had a working life, likely one that's largely behind us now. See what a story it has been! Not every episode was thrilling, with some chapters only fair to middling and others horrific. But it's unique and, as it unfolded, you smiled, supported, inspired, interacted and contributed to a greater purpose. In short, you made a difference. And that's all any of us can hope to do.

What to Do If You're
Facing Ageism at Work

- Know your own worth and don't engage with any ageism.

- Assess whether you want to stay where you are or whether a move somewhere else (or out on your own) might better serve you.

- Don't hold in your feelings. Talk them through with your friends because the chances are they've experienced something like this too.

- Try to handle it with grace, even if you go home and scream into a pillow.

- Remember that great phrase we encountered earlier: if you've been invited into the room, it's because you have a place in it, so own it.

Chapter Thirteen

Fern's Golden Rule: Never Put Anything in the Loft

*R*epowering means letting go of your stuff. Not everything – we all like the comfort of certain objects and pieces of clothing that mean something to us – but in general, we have a ton of items we don't need that someone else could enjoy. This is where the loft comes in. Did you fall for the insistence of a partner that all things could go in the loft? The problem is, the minute you put anything up there you'll want it back down again.

You're also unlikely ever to find anything interesting in a loft. The romantic notion that we'll stumble across a forgotten Monet or Picasso or great-granny's Fabergé egg collection is never going to happen. If we buy a house where the loft is full of the previous owners' stuff, it will invariably be nothing more interesting than a collection of rubbish records, some broken tools and a couple of rolls of unused insulation. I have bats in my loft, which is a far better option, as far as I'm concerned. I don't want to disturb them; they don't want to disturb me. All understood.

Step away from the loft!

Let's move on to the rest of the house now.

If your children have left home, then it's likely they will have left you a lot of their stuff that they didn't want to take with them but expect you to look after. But do you want to repurpose their old bedrooms and create a space for yourself? Here's how to do it.

Suggest that they come and sort through all their old schoolbooks, comic collections and warped tennis rackets ASAP, as they are now ready to be collected, or you're very happy to send them to the charity shop for them, if that would be helpful. I'm sure that will get them running over. It doesn't mean you won't have a spare bed for them when they do come to visit, it just won't be like their 'old' room.

Once their stuff has gone, you get the chance to turn it into a space that is just for you. The opportunities are endless. Think carefully about what sort of space you would like. Intoxicating, isn't it? My dream is to have an entirely white room that is completely empty; I can just go in there and lie on the floor and luxuriate in the peace and lack of anything that would annoy me or needs tidying or makes a noise. More practically, a craft room for sewing is Boo's choice. Two Cups has her own artist's studio … What would you like yours to be? If you want a ballet barre, put one in. If you want a writing room, create one. If you'd love a library, build some shelves and begin collecting books.

If you have more than one room not being used, your partner can have one too or (if you're clever) you could agree to him getting the bigger shed he's always wanted and you get to keep the second room. What a gift!

A sense of place is important to all of us. Having a home that just works is a real joy and privilege, and it can be an important step on your Repowering journey. My own house here in Cornwall is currently in the process of change but it's so fulfilling to see it taking shape. Especially when the Wellington boots in every size, kitchen gadgets used only once and sweaters that are full of moth holes are removed. Why did we hang on to it all? Over the years, I've both upsized and downsized several times. The one thing I know is true is that the more space you have, the more you'll fill. This house is half the size of the one I lived in before and it's crammed with stuff. But so was the previous one. If I moved to a mansion, it would be the same story.

My Cornwall home is feeling even more comforting and familiar now. When I come back on the train I always look out of the window as we cross the Isambard Kingdom Brunel bridge over the Tamar. As soon as we're on the other side of the river I have that feeling of *ahh, I'm home*. My house needs some work doing to it – new carpets, decorating, a reupholstered sofa – and I'm glad it's not stuck in aspic.

I like change and I enjoy putting my mark on it. I don't have to answer to anybody for what I'm doing and how I'm doing it. It's the freedom of not having to compromise.

Decorate your house exactly how you want it. This sounds like the most basic advice, but actually it needs to be said because for some reason we often seem to be scared to do what we really want and we end up with something bland. The horror of the judgement of friends and neighbours can push us towards the safety of boring. There was a phase recently of everyone painting everything in shades of grey. Why? I think it might be something to do with not scaring future buyers should we choose to move on. But it does show a lack of confidence in or a fear of colour. I love colour and my house is a mish-mash of many hues. Bright, bold, beautiful, exciting colours. I like pattern too. Mix them up. Clash them. If that sounds too scary (I do get it), try painting the inside of a cupboard in a bright shade. You'll smile every time you open the door.

Getting anything done at home is always a bit of an adventure. I had an electrician in once because the lights in the cooker hood wouldn't turn off. He fiddled about a bit, but the light was still there. Dimmer but definitely visible. When I asked him why that was, he said: 'Do you remember the dot you got in the middle of the screen when you turned your television off in the olden days?' I said I did. 'Well,' he continued, 'it's just like that – it's the residual electricity in the pipes.' Electricity in the pipes? Did he think I was a complete fool?

I am an absolute clutter-buck. If there's a shelf, I have to put something on it. If I run out of space, I'll put stuff on top of the things already on the shelf. Although I collect clutter, I'm a firm believer in having a place for everything and everything in its place. That way you can always find what you're looking for. The older I get, the more I forget where I've put everything. I cannot tell you how many precious things I have put somewhere safe and now can't find.

While my house is often a mess, there is order among the chaos. My desk drawer is full of bits and bobs, including paperclips, a ruler, rubber bands, a tape measure and my scissors and magnifying glass because I can't see without my glasses. I have my earpiece that I took every bit of television direction through. It was moulded to fit perfectly into my ear. Still got that – just in case.

I have had an office at home since I began writing. It was imperative to have somewhere I 'went to work'. In my previous house I had a tiny room upstairs, which was fine, but when I finally came to Cornwall I had a room that was the perfect space to write in, and I filled it with a lovely bookcase and some filing cabinets. It faces the garden and looking out the window often unlocks something in my mind when I'm struggling for inspiration.

Household budgets change when the children leave home and hopefully everything becomes a little bit less expensive. Food bills, energy bills, etc. Having said that, this whole cost of living crisis has probably put paid to that notion. You go and fill up with petrol and you wouldn't be surprised if they say, 'That's £500, please.' You nip into Tesco for a loaf of bread and a cucumber and it's £150. It's just crazy.

I have always written a money diary, a list of what comes in and goes out every month. I have them going back to the early 1980s. Now that inflation has gone bananas, I'm always in deficit. Every month. Everybody is. It's terrifying.

It's difficult to change our food shopping habits once the children leave home. We've been so used to buying for a family for years, so it's not surprising that it takes a while for our brains to catch up and realise things have changed. Shopping for one or two is entirely different from shopping for a family of four or six. One thing that's worked for me is to try to buy things that can be mixed and matched. I think of it a bit like managing a wardrobe. You look at a shirt and think, *I'll buy it because it goes with those trousers, that skirt, that jumper and those jeans.*

If you're on your own, or it's just two of you, like it is with Winnie and me, it's no longer necessary to do the big shop, which makes food-buying more of a pleasure and interesting. A little bit of this and that plus a treat. I have even enjoyed cooking more recently, trying out different recipes. Mind you, I bought a – very expensive – jar of preserved lemons the other day because they looked so beautifully exotic. I found a recipe for couscous with preserved lemon and mint. Sounded good. Then I saw that the lemons needed to be sliced, have all the innards scooped out and discarded, the remaining rind rinsed because the salt in the preserving liquid made them too salty, and then the rind cut into thin strips to add to the couscous. So much time, effort and expense for what? I could have just grated a lemon into the couscous for a few pence rather than the six quid the posh stuff cost me. What a racket! If you have some fruit, bacon, bread, eggs and cheese in, then there will always be something to eat.

My garden brings me great joy. If you find yourself with more time on your hands and you have a garden, I encourage you to get out more. People often think that a love of gardening comes with age, but for me it's been a lifelong pleasure. My mother was a keen gardener and would grow her own peas and beans among the roses and hollyhocks. There's nothing like eating peas fresh out of the pod, is there? It's an abiding memory from my childhood. She always kept the garden looking beautiful. She loved it. My father, too, was a good gardener, so maybe I've inherited green fingers.

When I bought my first house, which happened to be in Cornwall, in the early 1980s, it had a tiny garden but there was enough space for plenty of plants and I loved it. The garden I have now isn't big either. There used to be much more grass but I seem to have covered a lot of it in slate paving so I have somewhere for the table and chairs. Still, there's a flower called Mexican fleabane, or Erigeron, that still manages to foam through the cracks. I have abundant agapanthus, and their huge globe flowers bloom for weeks, a couple of ferns (of course), some clematis romping away over an arch and a herb garden, mostly tended by Winnie. It's like having another room. In the summer I put an all-weather rug down and put up a couple of umbrellas, and it's lovely to have somewhere nice to sit and eat.

I didn't have flowerbeds at all when I moved in because we're on bedrock here, so I asked a garden designer to create some raised beds in stone. Not just calf high but waist high, giving me the chance to future-proof my garden for years to come. No more bending down. They are wide enough that I can weed them from both sides and, because of their height, when I'm sitting in my office chair I am able to see the bright roses and delphiniums growing tall outside. Pretty and prac-tical! I may have started a trend?

I have an olive tree and a couple of apple trees, under which the bluebells flower in the spring. Winnie is also in the process of creating her own outdoor space, a decent-sized shed. She is an artist at heart, so it will be a great workspace for her to pursue her craft passion. It's still looking a bit like a building site – I need to paint it and weed outside – but the tulips and daffodils will come up around it, which will hide a multitude of sins.

This has been a big and, I feel, final home move for me. But it's never too late to move somewhere new. If you feel there's a home, a place on the planet where your heart is, why not do it? Or let out your own home and rent a place somewhere you've always wanted to go to test run it. It's worth living somewhere new for a calendar year so you can experience all the seasons. The winters here are windy, sometimes cold and often wet, but it's wonderful nonetheless. We have the sea and the beach, which belong to the locals once again. My daughters and I often go out with a flask and a pasty to sit on the rocks and watch the raging tide. People are often surprised that I'm 100 per cent based in Cornwall. I live here, work here, everything. They say, 'But surely not in the winter?' But, yes, I am here in the winter. The sense of community is what it's all about.

It's a privilege to live somewhere that people think is lovely enough to go to on holiday. I feel as if I'm permanently on holiday, but I do also scour the travel pages of the newspapers wondering where I might like to go to next.

The trouble is, as we get older, it's easy to make excuses not to do these things. I think, *Oh I can't leave the cats because I'll worry about them*, or *I can't go away in the summer because the garden is looking so lovely it would be a shame to miss it at its best and if I'm not here, who will keep on top of it?* We do this. We put handcuffs and leg irons on ourselves. The truth is, there are plenty of people I trust to look after the cats and the garden would be fine for a week or two.

If we want to travel, we must do it before it's too late. Do it while we're able enough to enjoy it. If you have cats, then, sure, they'll sulk a bit when you get back, but they love a good sulk. My indomitable stepmother, Jane, who has just turned 80, is a fearless traveller and an ex-travel agent. There's nowhere she hasn't been or can't tell you where the best hotels, restaurants and shops are. Every spring she takes a three-week break to travel to Thailand, dropping into Bangkok to go shopping and returning via any route that takes her fancy. She has the energy of a teenager. If she can do it, so can we!

We should talk about Repowering our social lives too. If you've had a life change, it's worth going back to the beginning and rediscovering what sort of social life you really want. Are you someone who really needs a busy social life? Are you unhappy if you're not out every night? Does a Saturday night in feel like the dullest thing ever or are you thrilled to get into your pyjamas with a good film? You'll find the route that works for you. If you're extrovert and you want to find a new, Repowered social life, it's all there for you. If you want a bit of socialising but not too much, then that's on offer too. The choice is yours and it's in your own hands.

And you can laugh together. All my friends make me howl. One of them, Jill, is always immaculately dressed. We often go for cocktails in Padstow. We talk about it as 'going for a waft' as we once went on a summer's evening and wafted around in our summer dresses. She looked around at all the young people staring at their phones and leant forward and whispered, 'They're all swiping on Tinder while all I do is swipe on Zara!'

Friends can truly help shape our *place*. They have the nimble ability to rekindle the marvellous stupidity, the hope and faith of our teenage years, when we were full of dreams and blessed with a sense of invincibility. It was an era when we took risks, believed in the impossible, and held an unshakeable faith in our future. True friends have a way of bringing this feeling back into our lives, no matter our age. They remind us of who we were before the weight of adult responsibilities and before life's inevitable ups and downs dimmed our enthusiasm. In their company, we often find the courage to dream big once again and embrace the joyous, silly moments that make life truly wonderful.

The lockdowns stopped us seeing many people and we haven't quite got back to full-throttle socialising yet. This is another area of life we need to Repower. When did you last invite friends over? It doesn't have to be anything grand. I'm not a very good cook, so I don't often have people over for dinner, but I'm good at afternoon tea with cakes and sandwiches. (Everybody enjoys a small cucumber sandwich!) No one comes to my house expecting a lavish feast, although I can roast a chicken nicely or a leg of lamb and I might be able to make a cottage pie.

Boo and Two Cups are great at getting friends over. Two Cups makes an exquisite sharing platter with little deli sausages, salamis, bits of cheese and wonderful grapes in amazing flavours like the candy floss ones. She makes it look like a painting. Boo makes incredible loaded nachos, which go down very well, with her famous Cosmos. In return for opening the odd garden show or compèring dog shows, I'm lucky enough to sometimes be gifted a bottle of champagne (unexpected and gratefully received!). I nearly always have one in the fridge for friends. A wonderful medicine for tears or laughter.

Some people find being a host is daunting, but you have to remember that the vast majority of other people at your table want you to succeed. And most people are way more worried about how they come across than they are about what you are saying or doing. Whenever I was nervous about what someone might think of me, my mother used to say, 'They're not looking at you because they're too busy looking at themselves.' If you're someone who is very nervous about social situations or making a mistake, take a deep breath and remember you're only human, and so is everyone else. In general terms, people are rooting for you and they are invested in your success. Don't make having friends over too complicated. Cook simply and remember your guests are not food critics. They have come to see you, have a laugh and enjoy themselves. I am such a bad cook that often I would suggest they brought some Rennies and I always serve Maltesers for pudding!

Start small: just asking someone over for a coffee is cheering when you feel a bit lonely, and remember to always ask about them and their lives so that you get to know them. Sharing stories builds trust and connection. Friends are wonderful things and as long as we have them, we'll always have a place in the world.

Modern Irritants

One of the great pleasures of life is inviting your friends over and spending all evening putting the world to rights over a bottle of wine. Nothing beats a good communal gripe about the modern world (in the privacy of your own home, of course, where no passing young people can raise their eyebrows at you condescendingly). Here are some of my (and your) top irritations. I want to thank my X and Instagram followers for their input here.

- Internet shopping is great but cardboard is not. It fights back when you fold it. And 'Please tear here' won't work with arthritic fingers. It's the next great invention, packaging that's easy to open for everyone.
- On the subject of packaging, when it comes to cotton buds, cut out the middleman and just throw them on the floor.
- Why are you never able to open a pill packet without it being the end with the folded instructions?
- QR codes – who thought these would be great for anything, especially restaurant menus? Instead of looking forward to conversation, we immediately have our heads buried in our phones.

- Being asked to 'rate our service' is the bane of life. No, I won't. Supposing we asked them to rate us as customers!
- No one loves a parking app.
- No one loves small print.
- Why don't shop assistants ask, 'How can I help you?' any more? Today they look up with a raised eyebrow and ask, 'All right?' The only answer from me is, 'Yes, I am fine, thank you.'

Chapter Fourteen

Coping with Loss

*M*ost of us don't reach our middle years without experiencing some form of bereavement. The death of someone close, the ending of a relationship, or the loss of a job. It is almost impossible to escape some form of sorrow. And there are so many other life events that can bring on a profound sense of grief.

I have been devastated when pets have died. I grew up with cats and I've always had an affinity with them. Back in the early 1980s, when I started my career at Westward Television in Plymouth, the job enabled me to buy my first little cottage in Cornwall. It needed a lot doing to it, which took some time and money, but eventually it was transformed into my dream home. All that was missing was a cat of my own. I put some feelers out and heard that there was a litter of kittens on a farm close by who were looking for a good home and that is how Wally (short for Cornwallis) came into my life. He was a handsome, affectionate, ginger boy and I adored him.

About a year later, I heard that another kitten needed rescuing. She was black and called Titch. The moment I saw her, I could see she had a mind of her own and, like many female cats, could be stroppy and overemotional (the cat lovers among you will understand!). The first thing she did was to ignore the name Titch. She hated it. One day, as she was tearing the sofa to shreds, she gave me a hard, telepathic stare and the name Delia popped into my head. This name she would answer to.

I used to get the bus to work and the cats would walk me to the point in the hedge where the bus stopped. Wally and Delia would see me off in the morning and would be waiting for me in the hedge when I got home at night. It felt special. One day, poor Delia, the cat who loved Maltesers and Christmas cake, died after being knocked down by a car. I was in London at the time, working on BBC *Breakfast Time* (as it was then called) on a try-out for a long contract. How I cried and cried. I still miss her.

I did get the job in London, so I had to sell my cottage and move up country. Maybe Delia's passing was a good thing as she never struck me as a London girl. Wally and I made the long journey up to my mother's house, where he stayed. She was good at taking in homeless animals. Wally lived there for many years until one day he just walked out of the house and disappeared. Cats often do that; they go off to die alone. I was inconsolable.

My mother was wonderful, and not just because she took in animals like Wally. She was a bit bohemian, gregarious and outgoing, and always accepted waifs and strays, human or otherwise, so we never knew who was going to appear for supper or lunch or what was going to happen next.

When my mother was newly divorced and single, she had to do everything she could to make ends meet. She took in lodgers, and she taught woodwork, art and drama at my first school, the small pre-prep school in Gerrards Cross where I got my reading cup, handily situated between Pinewood, Denham and Ealing film studios. The pupils were either very wealthy or the children of actors or directors.

One little boy loved telling tall tales. My mother overheard him talking to his friend about how high he could bounce on his space hopper. 'I bounced so high I went right over the roof of the house and into the front garden,' he boasted. His friend said, 'Oh, my dad does that in the helicopter.' It was that kind of school. My mother thought it hilarious. That was the brilliant thing about her: she found joy in the smallest – and most absurd – things.

She drove her beloved Triumph Herald – in Monaco blue, which she thought was very glamorous – and in the winter she'd wear a white *Dr Zhivago* fur hat.

One day, after we'd been to the dentist in Ealing, we were driving home on the A40. She would always ask me to light her cigarettes for her – I was about five and I loved doing it! Suddenly I noticed a man overtaking us, gesticulating wildly. But it wasn't because he was shocked at seeing a child with a cigarette in her hand – he was smiling at my mum because she was so striking.

She had lots of dates. She was attractive and funny and because she had experienced life-and-death situations during the war in the army, she had an enormous appreciation of life.

I adored her. As a single parent, she played such a central role in my life. Aged 94 when she died, she was still beautiful. She always dressed well and wore fabulous costume jewellery. I never once saw her without her bright red lipstick. She rarely complained, just accepted what life threw at her. Although she had a lot to deal with, she was always positive. Never too scared to do something. Never too nervous. I'm sure some parts of getting older were difficult for her, but it never showed.

She taught me that there are two ways of entering old age. You can bemoan all the things that have happened, play the victim and say: 'I'm not well. No, please don't be horrible to me. It's been a dreadful day.' Or you can declare, 'Well, today's been a bit of a bugger but I'm going to wake up tomorrow and it'll be over, and I'll still be alive.' We all have dual stories we could tell about our lives: how awful it has been or how wonderful it has been. The two narratives run parallel with each other. You cannot deny either of them but it's always better to think of the good times.

Before she died in 2018, my mother lived in a nursing home. For a long time, there was nothing wrong with her, mentally or physically. She'd had a new hip but other than that she was generally well. She just needed a bit of looking after. Unfortunately, whilst in the home she had a fall and broke her ribs, which punctured her lung. These two things led to her death. Although I was at the hospital when she died, I wasn't at her bedside. I was with my daughter Grace and my niece Rose, and we'd been with her all that morning as it was obvious she didn't have long left. We asked one of the nurses whether they could put her on a morphine shunt because she was in pain and her breathing was so laboured. They agreed and we were asked to leave the room. We went to the end of the corridor and as soon as we sat down, the nurse came running towards us and said, 'She's gone.'

Death is an intensely personal thing. It's my belief that it's something the person has to concentrate on to experience all that is happening to them. Maybe that is why so many people wait for their loved ones to pop out to the loo or get a cuppa. Don't be angry with them; they just needed to experience what was happening.

My mother grew up in in Malaysia, where there are many superstitions around death. So, when we got back into the room, I immediately said: 'We must open the windows and let her spirit go.' She looked so peaceful as we held her hand. She was still warm. I kissed her and then my sister arrived and put white roses on my mother's chest. We then sat in silence for a while after that.

Despite her death and the ensuing funeral, my mother still feels present in my life. I don't think I have grieved in the traditional sense. I had always dreamed of sailing to New York and back on a liner and, after her death, that's what I did, not least to give myself some quiet time in which to write. I could stare out of the window at the vast Atlantic for hours or go back to bed if I wanted. One evening I turned up for what I thought was the captain's cocktail party. In fact, it was a meeting of the choir and I thought, *Why not?* But when we started singing songs from *Les Misérables*, including 'Bring Him Home', I left in floods of tears because the lyrics are heartbreaking. The trip was cathartic, though, and afterwards I felt at peace. I don't think our body would give us the capacity for tears if they weren't for a purpose.

I am comforted by feeling my parents remain with me. Perhaps it's because I have a belief there is an existence after death. That it is not the end. I find the thought consoling and calming, and it gives me something to hold onto. And if, when I die, there is nothing, well, I won't know anyway.

We don't really talk enough about death. We deny it. Modern medicine is so incredible that we almost believe we will cheat death altogether. Dying is dying. It's going to happen and all we can do is hope it will be as peaceful and pain-free as possible. Discussing it openly sets a good template, especially for children. If you never talk about it, they won't know how to approach death.

Writing a will scares a lot of people, but actually it can be rather fun. I have written four and enjoyed changing it around, chopping people out and putting other people in, and thinking about where I want my belongings shared. My children know that they have equal shares. When I hear about families where one child gets more than another or one has been left out altogether, I feel so sad. In these situations, I don't think it's about the money. It's much more about the fact that the child will feel as though they were less loved.

If your family is a blended one, it can be harder. If at all possible, it makes sense to try to talk these things through with ex-partners so everyone is on the same page. Even if you don't agree with their plans (or they with yours), at least it will be something that can be talked about openly.

I mentioned earlier that you should ask your parents to grant you a lasting power of attorney (LPA), so that you can help them make decisions, or make them on their behalf if they're no longer capable of doing so. If you haven't done so already, you should also get one set up yourself for your own partner or children, or whoever you trust to help you if you need assistance in managing your finances or health care in the future. Whoever you choose must be 18 or over, and you need to discuss it with them first so they understand the responsibilities involved. You can have as many attorneys as you like. Bear in mind that you might think your spouse or partner will automatically be entitled to make decisions about your finances or care if you're incapable, but that's not the case – you still need to have set up an LPA.

There's an assumption that writing a will or setting up an LPA is something that only the elderly need to do, but that isn't true. Sure, the chances of becoming incapacitated increase the older we get but we never know what's around the corner. In 2016, I had sepsis and was extremely ill. I'd had a hysterectomy and was home after a couple of days. As I left, the nurses gave me a number to ring if I had any problems. Within about 48 hours I was in tremendous pain. I rang in the middle of the night and they told me to take some painkillers. I did and it got a little better. Over the coming days, though, I went up and down until I suddenly plummeted.

We called for an ambulance twice during that week and the emergency workers were wonderful but each time, when I spoke to the paramedics, I declared that I was fine and didn't need to go hospital. I felt a bit of a fraud when they arrived; surely I would get better soon? No one mentioned sepsis. Eventually things got even worse and I rang my doctor's surgery the next day, where the receptionist said she'd get the doctor to ring me. It was much later by the time the doctor called and by that point I was in so much pain I could barely speak and my breathing was very shallow.

The doctor said: 'Is it to do with your gastric band?'

I said: 'What? No, that was eight years ago! I've just had a hysterectomy!'

Once again, the advice was to take some painkillers. I was in bed, lying face down and trying to hold my tummy. It felt as if I was having bad contractions. Then suddenly a feeling of calm washed over me and I thought, *I'm dying. That's what's happening here. I'd rather die now because this is too much*. And then – and I don't quite know how this happened – an ambulance arrived. Paramedics wrapped me up and off I went.

I was wheeled into resus. Some doctors came in looking worried. There was a big sign on the wall saying, 'Could it be sepsis?' And it suddenly clicked in my head: that's what was wrong.

The gynaecologist who delivered Grace heard I was in the hospital and came down to see me. She was a senior consultant so afterwards all the staff joked, 'Oh, you have some good contacts!' They gave me stronger painkillers, which was a great relief, and then took me off for an x-ray and a scan. Grace wheeled me down in a wheelchair. I couldn't get up onto the table as my stomach was in so much pain. When the results of the x-ray came back, they showed my abdomen was full of abscesses. I was given lots of antibiotics and an operation was scheduled for the next day.

The consultant who was looking after me this time was brilliant. Her name was Geraldine. She told me she was going to try to aspirate the abscesses without having to open me up. She was with a male surgeon who listened, then said: 'And when that fails, I'm going to open you up from here to here and then here to here.' He mimed an action across my abdomen that resembled a hot cross bun. 'And cut out the abscesses and clean all the poison. Of course, the poison will spread through your body, so you're going to be ill for a long time.'

When he listed all the drugs I would have to take after the operation, I was terrified. He then said to Geraldine, the consultant: 'I think we'll be all right.' And I said: 'Geraldine will definitely do it right.'

Phil and Grace were in the room as a nurse prepared me to go to theatre. She asked if I wanted her to put a plaster over my wedding ring or to take it off. I handed it to Grace. When I talked to her about it later, she said: 'I know you gave it to me because you wouldn't want it taken off your dead finger!'

I believed wholeheartedly that I was dying but I wasn't frightened. I knew everything would be all right. I remember lying in the room where they give the anaesthetic, looking at the clock and thinking, *I thought I had a bit more life left, but there you go*. The anaesthetist was talking to me about cycling. I thought, *Blimey, my last conversation is going to be about bloody cycling*, and as the anaesthetic went in, I thought, *This is it, that's me done*. It wasn't though. I woke up in the recovery room.

Geraldine came in the next morning and said: 'I wasn't able to sleep last night because I was thinking about you. I think we're going to have to go in again.' I replied: 'No you're not. I'm going to be fine. I really am.' And from then on, I rallied.

I hadn't eaten for about ten days because I was feeling so ill. Then one evening Winnie came in with Phil and was munching her way through a bag of flame-grilled steak crisps with ridges. Oh my God! It took me five minutes to eat just one but it was the best thing I've ever tasted.

It took about two years to recover and get my strength back, but my brush with death left me oddly calm. I think it's because I have thought about my own death often and talked about it with the children. When my final journey is over, I will be popped in the local churchyard, which is a special place.

It's not only death that leaves us grieving. The end of a friendship brings with it incalculable sadness. There was one that hit me hard. It wasn't that our lives had taken different courses and we'd simply drifted apart. This ending felt way more brutal. This was a girlfriend I was extremely fond of and, suddenly, something – and I still don't know quite what – happened and the shutters came down for her. She wouldn't connect with me or speak to me at all. It is mystifying and it hurt but that's her choice. We can never know what goes on in someone else's mind and if they no longer wish to maintain a relationship, we must accept that decision.

The loss of a job or facing a major career setback can be a source of deep grief, too. Often our work is tied to our identity and our sense of purpose. Losing it can shake us to the core. Uncertainty can lead to anxiety, even if the job at stake isn't an especially good one. It's more than just the job; it's the colleagues you've been working with, the lifestyle and perhaps even the routine. Like most people, I enjoy routine. It's comforting to know what is going to happen next, but I am nimble enough to handle change too.

Some people are enveloped with a sense of sorrow around ageing. It can be tough at times. I know first-hand that your sixties, for example, can beckon in frailties where none previously existed. An illness, a sudden injury, or the gradual decline of physical or mental abilities can trigger a profound sense of loss. I depend on my spectacles, which is irritating because I keep losing them or they are always upstairs when I am downstairs, or vice versa. I have also started wearing hearing aids after my hearing diminished due to wearing an earpiece for 40-odd years at work. The aids are tiny and invisible, which is great until you lose one.

Often people can't wait to retire and make endless plans about all the exciting things they're going to do. I am addicted to holiday brochures. I'm not retired yet, but I am trying to prepare for the feeling when the phone finally stops ringing. It's perfectly natural though and we must give ourselves time to process any big change.

We may miss the daily routine of our working life or even the noise, chaos and fun that our children take with them when they leave. I love having Winnie at home and Grace living just ten minutes away. I adore how included their friends make me feel. They walk in chorusing, 'Hello, Fernie B. How are you, Fernie B?'

We can also lament missed opportunities and unfulfilled dreams. Perhaps it's a career path we never pursued, a relationship that never blossomed, or a life goal that seems increasingly out of reach. It happens often to women at menopause, the mourning of fertility. Which is odd because a baby is probably the last thing they'd want and they're often thrilled that their children are older and more independent. It's just hard, I guess, when these decisions are taken out of our hands. Younger people talk a lot about collective grief. A loss of security that comes with global events such as climate change, the pandemic and the relentless horror of war.

We must accept that grief is a normal part of being human. That we get attached to people, places and things.

A cliché, I know, but it's the price we pay for love. I'm lucky in that I'm generally pragmatic and I try to look on the bright side all the time. Sometimes I wonder if it's my brain tricking me when perhaps what I need to do is to sit down and say, 'This is sh*t and I need to stop.' But something pushes me through and I find myself thinking, 'Come on, this'll be all right.'

A good exercise to try at any age, but certainly when you're older, is to flip through your photo albums. It always brings with it a great deal of joy and some sorrow. Pictures might feature those who have hurt you. This is the time to look at those photos. Remember what was going on and then look at their face and forgive them (… and then maybe rip it up!). Forgiveness doesn't mean you have to let someone back into your life, but it will be a load off your shoulders. A weight you don't have to carry through life.

I have been lucky in that I have never fallen apart with grief. I've said goodbye to two marital homes now and, looking back, it was no hardship. It was much easier to say, 'It's fine,' knowing I can go on and create something nicer, better, calmer. I've moved around quite a lot and have a bit of a ritual when it comes to leaving a house. Once it's emptied, I clean it to the best of my ability and, of course, I make sure there are loo rolls and working lightbulbs. Then I walk around the house and thank all the rooms for the happy times I've spent in them.

That doesn't mean change is easy. It's hard for most of us. So now is the time to box clever, to anticipate it and negotiate with our emotions on the change that's coming. We don't have to make any big decisions immediately. I'm a great fan of setting aside some time to have a little think. Time spent on reflection and self-reflection is never wasted. After we've given ourselves this cost-free luxury, we're way more prepared and can make decisions in a less emotional, more practical way.

Opening Up to Others

It's all too easy to start getting introspective if you are grieving for something or someone. To live in your own head, looking inward, judging yourself and others. But there are antidotes at hand.

- Do something for someone else. Help out. Volunteer. Offer lifts. Do someone's garden. And listen, listen, listen to their story.

- Be true to yourself and celebrate the wisdom, age and person you are. The more comfortable you are in your skin, the more approachable you will be to others.

- Don't keep family secrets. The next generation need to know their history. I'm glad I found mine at 55 but I wish I had known it sooner.

- Remember that, after love, time is the most precious gift we can give and receive.

Chapter Fifteen

Challenge Yourself

I never want to stop having adventures, even when there's jeopardy. I really believe that age is just a number and that it shouldn't stop us doing exactly what we want. Who has the right to say that a woman in her sixties shouldn't wear a bikini? Or that a woman in her late sixties shouldn't travel on her own to remote destinations? Or that we should have a prim haircut and wear sensible shoes? No one. That's who. We should do exactly what we want to do when we want to do it. Who would we offend by being ourselves? Of course, we need to take care that our actions don't hurt anyone, but other than that, the world really is open to us to do whatever we want to.

When I was in my mid-fifties, and the boys were coming up to 18, the conversation turned to tattoos. I wasn't completely against the idea, but I didn't want them to do it just because they were 18 and they could. It needed more thought than that. So I hatched a plan to put them off for now. I would get a tattoo. If your 52-year-old mum has a tattoo, it's suddenly not so cool any more. Plus I could tell them how much it hurt.

I made an appointment at a tattoo parlour in Marlow and asked for two butterflies on my left hip. When I returned home, the boys hadn't got back from school yet, so I showed my husband what I had done. He went quiet. 'It's as if I don't know you at all. You're like a stranger.' When the boys got home, I told them and they were only mildly surprised. On their 18th birthday only one of them got inked, so my plan half worked.

A few years later, I was filming a programme for Easter in Jerusalem for the BBC. It was an amazing place to visit. One of the places I went to was a shop where a family has been tattooing pilgrims for generations. They use the same olive wood stencils that have been used since the 16th century. In those olden days, coming to Jerusalem on pilgrimage was an important step in one's religious life. As a memory and physical sign they had been there, the pilgrims would get a tattoo, often on their wrist or arm, so that on the road home, when they shook hands with strangers who were on their own pilgrimage, it would be known that they were a friend, not a foe. It felt so right, after hearing that story, that I should have one too.

In the tattoo parlour I watched as a woman and her two grown-up daughters each had a tiny cross tattooed on their wrist. So simple. When it was my turn, I asked for the same. I could see the director's face and she was looking a little concerned, but when I offered my wrist, the man said, 'Yes, of course, of course.' So, I had it done on camera. The director worried that I might be contravening a health and safety rule and asked me, 'Are you sure? We're not coercing you into doing this. The BBC are not forcing you.' In minutes it was done. Painless.

It has faded now but you can still see the outline faintly. Curiously it's one of those things that I am most asked about and I have to lift my sleeve to prove it's still there. One day I shall return to Jerusalem and have it re-inked, but I would have to go back to the same man so it would remain authentic.

The tattoo serves to remind me that, although I'm not a perfect Christian, I do have faith. That doesn't mean I don't worry about things. Of course I do. In fact, I can make anything into a worry if I think about it long enough. The trick, though, is that I recognise that and I don't allow it to stop me doing what I must do, should do or will do.

Looking back to my youth, I realise I have always had an adventurous spirit. I was the person who would always say yes to a dare. Perhaps that's why I decided to enter the *Celebrity Big Brother* house in 2024. An adventure was beckoning.

When the call came through, I surprised myself by not saying no immediately. My agent Dylan Hearn is a calm man with a cool head. We had a logical conversation one day where he laid the plan out to me. He reckoned that I could either be the most hated woman in Britain, the most loved woman in Britain or simply lost in the melee. I would not win (because although older people watched, younger people voted), but would probably survive the first eviction and be out by the end of the second week. Excellent advice and strategy, so on the basis that I understood all that, I thought, *Why not?* The timing felt right. I didn't want anything from it other than an adventure and I had nothing to lose.

I wasn't allowed to tell anyone that I was going into the *Big Brother* house, except for my children. It was important to me that I was able to talk to them about it, because if one of them had said to me, 'No, Mum, don't,' I wouldn't have done it. But they all said, 'Of course, Mum, go for it!' So I went for it.

In the meeting a few weeks beforehand, I asked the producer what was the worst thing I could expect, and she said it would be the boredom. She wasn't wrong. That started even before filming as we were taken away to individual hotel rooms and kept in purdah for 36 hours before making our big entrance. We had no books, telephones or televisions and as a result our minds were scrambled before the audience clapped eyes on us. I think this was done so that we would be desperate for conversation once we entered the *CBB* house.

Our sole task at the hotel was to empty our suitcases and re-pack everything into a set of three special *CBB* ones. They were very chic and we even got to keep them at the end, which we were thrilled about. We had already been told that we were not allowed to wear stripey clothes, because these can cause a strobe effect on television, and that we couldn't have anything with logos on. A member of the production team would then come along to check that the clothes we'd packed followed their guidelines. This wasn't my first rodeo on TV, so I thought the stripes I'd chosen would be fine as they weren't too narrow. They weren't fine. I had to get rid of three pairs of trousers, a bunch of T-shirts and a shirt. So, I lost 50 per cent of my wardrobe before I even went in! Our remaining clothes were then catalogued by the production team, down to the last pair of knickers. We also had to hand over any medication. (Once we were in the house, we were given our own personal lockers in the room where the washing machines were, and we would find our medication dispensed in there each day.)

We each had a chaperone assigned to us to make sure we behaved whilst we were in the hotel and didn't leave our rooms. They would go down to collect our meals and when mine left, I thought I'd turn the TV on to pass the time, which was when I discovered that it had been disconnected and there was literally nothing to do.

On the afternoon we were due to start filming, I had my hair and make-up done by the glam squad, who aren't allowed to talk to you, and then at 3.30pm, my suitcases containing everything I had with me were taken away. So there I was, sitting in my room, in my dress, make-up done, waiting on my own for hours. Eventually, someone came to collect me, and I was whisked through the hotel, swathed by umbrellas, to stop anyone recognising who I was. There was a Mercedes waiting outside with blacked-out windows which took me to the studios in North West London, where we parked up. Over the wall I could just see the beam of the arc lights and hear the cheers of the crowds.

We were all given a code name to help maintain secrecy and so emails about us couldn't be tracked. Mine was 'Finland'. On the radio, there were messages about other contestants. 'Berlin has entered the house,' I heard the radio crackle, and wondered who on earth that might be. The driver remained quiet. Even he was barred from talking about the show.

After waiting for about an hour, another, even bigger, Mercedes pulled up and I changed cars. This time I was only driven for a matter of metres before reaching the steps. It had been raining and the stairs were slippery and my skirt too long, but I made it. The audience were lovely and cheering and the hosts AJ Odudu and Will Best were there waiting with a big hug. My heart was in my mouth as I made my way to the door and I thought, *What am I doing?!* I turned round and waved before walking through the doors, which shut behind me. I was the last one in, so everyone was already there.

Earlier in this book, we touched on confidence and the example of getting over your fears in a party situation. This was a prime example of that. Everyone was smiling and trying to look the happiest and wanting to be liked. We were all wanting to get on together. And curiously, we did! There weren't factions, as far as I was aware.

Once inside, there was often nothing to do. We were kettled and unsettled at every turn. Some days, when there weren't tasks, the programme makers would close off selected rooms, to corral us into either the bedroom, the kitchen/dining-room area or the garden. This was clever because it forced us to talk to each other and invent silly games. Food was rationed and used as a motivator, to win the games. If we won, we got a double budget, or if we lost, we would get nothing and the fridge would be emptied overnight. There was no dishwasher and only a small sink, but at least there was a washing machine and tumble drier. The bedroom was huge with tall ceilings, but of course the whole *Big Brother* house is within another building, so there was no sunshine and you couldn't open the windows to get fresh air. It did feel claustrophobic at times. Little did I know that I would be there for 19 nights. If I'd known that, I might not have agreed to go in!

The programme makers were diligent about everyone's physical and mental health, though. All the housemates were seen by a doctor and psychotherapist a few weeks before filming and there was always a psychotherapist watching the live feed, so if someone was looking lonely or upset or not engaging with the others, they'd call them to the diary room to make sure they were OK. We could ask to talk to the psychotherapist at any time, and I discovered that most of us had at some stage. You would arrange a time to go into the diary room where you would speak to the psychotherapist through the camera. It felt safe and secure in that room and a comforting voice would speak back to you, instantly making you feel calm. During that time, they cut the microphone and camera from recording, so it's just between you and the psychotherapist. I felt very taken care of.

We knew we had to be careful about what we said as we were always being recorded. For example, if we talked about certain subjects, forgetting the cameras were on us, that would not be in the edit. Of course, I forgot about the cameras watching everything and I forgot that what I might be saying would be heard by everyone. Of course I did!

A lot of it was hard and I know I seemed to cry a lot, but I wasn't sad, it was just a lot to process. In the end, I was up for every eviction and each time I looked forward to seeing my family. What I didn't know was that they had to be at the studio for EVERY eviction! On the penultimate eviction, we were allowed an on-camera rendezvous with a loved one for just a few minutes, and Winnie came. I was sitting on a bench for ages, but finally we were reunited. She reassured me by saying three things: 'You're not snoring, the cats are OK and you haven't been embarrassing.' So that was a relief! I had no idea that she, Two Cups and my agent were close by almost all the time, sometimes even looking at me through the two-way mirrors in the camera traps. They became friendly with all the crew, who I didn't ever meet. When I finally got out (last woman standing and all the way to the final!), they were exhausted and far more stressed than me. While Two Cups and Winnie were living it up in London, waiting for my eviction, Boo was tethered to Cornwall, keeping the home fires burning and making sure that Dr Ian Mackerel, Barbara and Lady Silky Paws remained fed and tickled. See? She is the very definition of a good friend.

I'm grateful to all the people who picked up the phone and voted for me. It took me a couple of weeks on the outside to realise that people were keeping me in right up to the end. That was incredible. There was one point when Dylan, my agent – with his head in his hands – thought: *Oh f**k, she's going to win!*

I'm still computing it all, but it was worth the risk because it was a grand adventure. What makes me laugh most now is people coming up to me to tell me that they never usually watch *Big Brother* as it's rubbish and then they go on to remember all of the things I said or did.

When it comes to Repowering, this was a pretty extreme example. You don't need to tackle something huge straight away; sometimes it's better to start off small. You will know what feels right for you.

When I was in my mid-forties, I decided to get my motorbike licence. I have always liked things with an engine. Phil had a motorbike and I used to ride pillion. Thrilling! Taking the test would make me a better car driver, he told me. (He was right!) I started small, riding a moped with an L-plate for a television programme where I had to become a dispatch driver for a day around East Sussex. Such a speed freak was I that a man on a push bike overtook me ... The upshot was that I did my CBT (compulsory bike test), which meant I could ride on the roads with an L-plate, then I had a set of lessons before taking the test and ... I passed!

Phil was waiting for me, so I pulled a disconsolate face and he was quick to comfort me. 'Don't worry,' he said. 'It took me two goes before I got my licence.' He didn't believe me when I told him I'd passed, until I produced the piece of paper that proved it. I proceeded to buy a Honda CB500 motorbike, which was fun, but hopeless for doing a weekly shop: no boot! Then I fell pregnant with Winnie and I came to my senses. My motorbiking days were over. Ah, but maybe one day?

A few years later, I gave in to the need for speed again, this time on the water. I mentioned earlier my love of boats. Well, I chose to take a Level Two Powerboat course. This means you can call me skipper if we're on a rib – and I find that totally thrilling! I love boats. Not yachts because I'd get seasick, but a boat with an engine. The kids know I love the speedboats at Padstow so I've told them to take my ashes on one last trip around the bay, on a speedboat all lit up with fairy lights.

My lessons took place in Rock, just over the water from Padstow. I'd been taught the basics – how to beach the boat, how to get it onto a buoy, how to guide it back into a dock, and how to pull a man back after he's fallen overboard – all with an instructor. On the day of the test, as I'd been taught, I checked the weather and the tide, I told someone the time we were going out and where I planned to go. With all my planning done, I ticked off the list and got into the boat with my tutor. I was nervous to start with, but he seemed confident and confidence breeds confidence. I was all ready to get underway.

I was a little worried at the mouth of the Camel Estuary because there's a sandbank called the Doom Bar, a treacherous hazard for boats said to have been created by a mermaid's dying curse, and it's easy to get lodged on it when the tide is low. Happily, we managed to get over it – although it was a bit touch and go – and then we were out to sea, speeding around the tiny offshore islands. It was exhilarating. I concentrated on everything I'd been taught. I looked out for lobster pots and fishing lines and drove alongside the waves so as not to be turned over. I practised my 'man overboard' procedure and beaching. Eventually, we came back to shore and I looked at him with such anticipation. He just smiled and said: 'You passed as soon as you went over the Doom Bar.'

It was such a thrill. Such a confidence boost. It made me feel as if I could do anything. So, take my advice: if there's something you'd love to do, then go out and do it. Embrace the challenge, because who knows where it might lead.

I mentioned earlier that when I was in my late forties, I realised all my time was either spent at work in a television studio, at home or in the Co-op. That was literally my life. There was nothing else. Every second of it was full and there wasn't a moment that was just mine, not even on the loo. Don't get me wrong, those years were wonderful, but – as anyone who's had four children under ten will tell you – a working mum's life never stops. Life takes on the inevitability of Groundhog Day. Work, home, supper, bath, story, bed. Repeat.

It was around that time I saw an advertisement in a newspaper with a picture of Professor Robert Winston, the well-known fertility expert. As the mother of IVF twins, I was aware of his work. I'd also interviewed him several times on *This Morning*. The ad, which featured a picture of the professor complete with his marvellous moustache, was looking for women to cycle along the banks of the Nile in Egypt to raise funds for his charity, linked to the Genesis Research Trust. It was a spoof of the First World War poster with General Kitchener pointing and saying, 'Your country needs you', but instead it said, 'Professor Winston needs you.' It was effective as it got me wondering, *Why does he need me?* and that was the start of some wonderful years as patron of his charity, Genesis Research Trust, which raised money by cycling all over the world.

I've always cycled and I love it. As a child I would disappear off on my bike for hours. I adored the freedom of it, and the independence it offered. It made me feel as if I could go anywhere and do anything. Repowering, for me at least, really does involve going back to the past and trying to reconnect with bits of myself that have got crushed under the weight of adult life. When I saw the advert, I knew I had to do it. What could be more freeing than being on two wheels again?

I also loved the idea of doing something with a group of women, as well as having no responsibilities for a week other than to take care of myself and get the miles in. Winnie was at nursery. Grace and the boys were at school. There was nothing stopping me except work.

I put in my request for a week off and later my boss asked, 'Where are you off to?' I think she imagined I'd be lounging by a pool somewhere, not taking on a huge challenge like this. I told her I was going on a 400km charity bike ride up the Nile. And, before I knew it, she made plans for a camera crew to follow my journey. Not only that, she organised a competition for two *This Morning* viewers to take on the 'Challenge of a Lifetime' and join me. They had to write in and explain why they wanted to challenge themselves. It would be brilliant for raising awareness but maybe not quite the peaceful trip I was expecting. But by God it worked out well.

I was 47ish. I wasn't at my fittest or my lightest and I was totally out of practice when it came to cycling. But even planning the trip gave me back a part of myself I'd been missing. It wasn't just the idea of the adventure. It was the thought of pushing myself out of my comfort zone. So I began training in earnest six months before the ride. *This Morning* introduced me to my personal trainer, Julie Dawn Cole, who played Veruca Salt in the original *Charlie and the Chocolate Factory*. On our training rides, she would regale me with stories of filming, which kept me going.

Finally, the day came to meet up with all the other participants at the airport. We were easy to spot. It's not difficult to identify a group of nervous-looking women with cycle helmets attached to their rucksacks. We met as strangers and ended as friends. The flight to Cairo went smoothly and we were transferred to our hotel easily. Our hotel was actually a Nile cruise ship. Unlike any other subsequent trip, we had the luxury of the same bed every night. No packing and unpacking.

The first morning I looked out of the window of my cabin and saw a squadron of bikes glinting in the sun outside. This was getting real. The trip was to take us down to the

Aswan Dam and then back up again. We were to see all the temples and sights along the way, including the Valley of the Kings. Every morning we'd leave the boat and every evening the boat would be waiting for us at the next stop.

Some of the terrain we would encounter was much hillier than you would imagine, and the extremes of heat were surprising. During the day, cycling through the desert, it was topping 40 degrees, but as soon as the sun sank, we felt the chill and pulled on our jumpers. It seemed we were miles from civilisation and then suddenly we'd catch a glimpse of a man standing by the side of a sandy track and we'd be completely bemused by where he could have come from. But mostly, when I looked to the horizon, there would be nothing. I'd pass the hollowed-out dead bodies of camels lying by the side of the road. I could see their ribs with the skin still on them. It felt extraordinary, almost biblical. I felt as if I'd travelled more than 2,000 years back in time.

Part way through the 400km ride I really thought I couldn't bear another minute. It was gruelling. What drove me on was the voice of my cousin in my head saying, 'You'll never do it.' In response, a different part of me thought, *I'll show you.* I was also inspired by the women around me. I'd look at them and know they were feeling the same way. Team spirit kicked in. We spurred each other on.

Since that initial ride I've cycled all over the world with that core group of women I met on the trip. Among other destinations we've been to Cuba, Panama, Costa Rica, Nicaragua, Vietnam, Cambodia, Russia, Estonia, India, Sri Lanka, Zanzibar, Tanzania, Madagascar and China. We've done around 14 rides in all and raised millions for charity.

I managed to achieve so much on that bike but I've never really appreciated it until now. At the time, Repowering wasn't a concept I was thinking of as a way of life, but that's what I was doing. I remember every last ounce of energy the girls and I put into it. Looking back, I remember the many great experiences I've had and how many amazing women I've met.

On the first ride they didn't expect me to do the whole thing. I think they thought I'd just turn up with full make-up and a camera crew, cycle long enough to be filmed and then get back into some luxury air-conditioned limo. They'd say things like, 'Fern, we didn't expect you to be sitting with us in third class on the plane,' or 'We didn't expect you to be sleeping in the desert on a camp bed without any water.'

There is nothing – and I repeat nothing – remotely chic about cycling. The uniform is as unglamorous as it gets. You can't wear knickers because they rub, so padded shorts are *de rigueur*. There's a breathable cycling shirt, shoes with cleats, socks and a bra. The shirts we always wore advertised the charity and the specific ride we were on.

The lack of glamour was a big part of it for me. I wanted to experience it fully, in all its horror. That's the gung-ho, up-for-anything part of me. I love mucking in and being part of a team. You're much more likely to hear me say, 'Yes, I'll dig a latrine!' than you are to find me walking a red carpet. That's way scarier to me.

Every cycling trip we undertook was amazing. Jordan stands out. It was hot, more than 40 degrees Celsius. But the great thing about being on a bike is you make your own breeze as you cycle. When we arrived at our camp, in the middle of the desert in a place called Robert's Rock, the Bedouins had built a fire for us. We were all desperate to wash. When you get that hot and sweaty, if you don't wash and get into dry clothes, you become susceptible to nappy rash. Of course, the Bedouins had no bath to offer us, but they had a long trough with four taps. I was so desperate to be clean that I took off almost all my clothes and washed naked in the middle of the desert. I just didn't care. Modesty becomes totally meaningless at times like that. I do slightly blush when I remember the Bedouins looking at us mad women stripping off and standing there showing our arses.

They didn't say anything, though, and cooked us delicious food. I remember sitting watching the sparks from the fire in the dark, feeling incredibly happy and extremely tired. It was such a pure feeling. Then we went to sleep under the stars among the camels, and I snored and kept everyone awake!

The next day we headed for an enormous mountain. We got to a point where there was an opportunity to split off. The elite could carry on up this long and high climb to the village right at the top of the mountain, or there was the option of getting in the minibus and being driven up. I got in the minibus with several others, marvelling at the courage of the girls continuing to cycle. It took them two hours to get to us. It was brilliant when they got there. We cheered them in and spent the whole of lunch telling them how proud we were that they'd done it, and the team spirit soared.

The cycle ride down was amazing. It felt as if it were three hours of not having to push the pedals once. At the end of every ride (which is usually five days long) there is a finish line and a medal ceremony. And then it's off to have a lovely cold beer!

There's something marvellously triumphant about the end of a long ride, wherever it is. In India, we went from Agra to Jaipur. I fell in love with India and desperately want to return. One night we slept in a crumbling palace and another in white tents right out of the Raj. The tent I was sharing even had a small bathroom at the back – a china loo sitting on the sand. I tried it before realising that it wasn't plumbed to anything! On the way home we had to get a train from Jaipur to Delhi and there were literally cockroaches falling off the ceiling. In fact, now I come to think of it, cockroaches were a big part of every ride we did that trip. It got to the point where if there were only two cockroaches under my pillow, that was luxury!

When we got to Delhi, we were taken to a hotel that was literally a knocking shop. Some of the rooms had seven beds.

Some had no beds. We had another two lovely 'Challenge of a Lifetime' winners with us on this trip and I was feeling awful that these poor women were stuck in the hotel from hell, so I made the decision to get us out of there. I said to them: 'Right, girls, we're not staying here, you're coming with me.' We found an award-winning hotel, The Oberoi, which had Italianate marble bathrooms, teak floors and wide beds with crisp, white cotton sheets. We walked in, stinking, at two o'clock in the morning, and the staff were wonderful. They found us beautiful rooms with the softest of pillows and sparkling bathrooms. My bottom was so sore from cycling, it was like the worst kind of nappy rash. I had a bath and when I got out I glanced at my bum in the mirror. It was red raw.

We all had our doors open so we could call to each other down the corridor and we were ordering gin and tonics. I couldn't have these poor ladies whom we'd inveigled to come and have 'the challenge of your life' sleeping in that awful hotel. They'd invested a lot in the ride and one of them couldn't tolerate spicy food so was constantly hungry. So, that last night was my treat.

Cycling in China sounded great on paper. We were to start in Beijing and ride to the Great Wall of China. Unfortunately, the weather was against us. For almost the entire trip, we were in cold, wet cloud. The high spot (literally, because we climbed a steep road) was arriving in a village where we had an incredible Chinese lunch. It was magical and the food was delicious.

Another notable cycling trip was the Challenge 57. It got its name because I did it in my 57th year and we cycled roughly 57 miles a day. The trip began in John O'Groats and ended up in Land's End. We travelled up on the sleeper train and were picked up in a van from Inverness station. Then it was another two or three hours by road to get to John O'Groats. Sitting in the van, I remember thinking, *Gosh, this is the last time I'm going to look through a windscreen for three weeks.*

Around 20 of us did the whole distance while others joined us for various legs. It took 20 days, including two rest days. Spring unfolded in front of us as we travelled south from Scotland. Suddenly we'd turn a corner and there would be drifts of snowdrops or a deluge of daffodils.

For some reason the idea of travelling from Scotland to Cornwall can make it feel as if it will be all downhill. It is certainly not. For a start, it took us almost a week to get out of Scotland, where there were some steep climbs, and second, the prevailing winds were in our faces rather than at our backs.

We stayed in a mix of youth hostels and hotels. When we got to Shap Fell in the Lake District, it was blowy. The high open hill left us vulnerable as the gale was so strong it was lifting women off their bikes. So we had to dismount, lie on our bikes and wait to get rescued.

It went quite smoothly from then on though, and when we got into Cornwall, I remember thinking, *Hey, I'm home now, this is fine.* But Cornwall was the worst part of the journey. It was so hard and so hilly, crossing Dartmoor. Nevertheless, arriving at Land's End felt like a glorious achievement. Despite all the far-flung places I'd visited for exotic cycling adventures, this was the most life-enhancing trip I'd ever done. Cycling has brought so much into my life. It began as a way to Repower when I needed to reclaim some of myself when I was juggling motherhood and an exhausting work schedule and it has – on and off – kept me going ever since. It brings me back to myself when I am feeling a little unanchored.

When I did my first ride, I remember thinking, *I hope my kids are proud of me.* But 20 years on I'm not sure it's at the forefront of their memories of me. But still, at some point, I want them to say, 'My mum – she was 47 and she did it!'

Even now, well into my sixties, I don't feel like giving up cycling any time soon. In fact, I'm doing a trip again later this year, a chance to catch up with some bike buddies, to chat and laugh and eat and loll in a spa. We're 20 years older than we were back then, so we'll have electric bikes this time. We have nothing to prove!

There are so many things we can do to get out of a slump. Raising money for charity has always been an inspiration for me. And, honestly, there are a billion things all of us can do for a good cause if we want to, whether it's sitting in a bath of baked beans or climbing Kilimanjaro. My motto is *just do it*. Whether it's a tattoo in the Holy Land or 100km a day on a bike in 40°C heat.

Embrace that new longing to explore the world and rediscover yourself. Who you used to be. Who you are now. Who you want to be. Find your lost self.

The Route to Repowering

Cycling hundreds of miles in a desert is just one way to Repower but it doesn't have to be a big adventure to make us feel that the future is there for the taking. Older, creakier, wiser we may be, but we still have the energy for Repowering. Here are some points to consider:

- Take up a new hobby. Consider a career change. Draw up a life plan with signposts showing where you want to go.

- Look at yourself! You're incredible and don't tell me you're not.

- It's been a hot wash on a fast spin, but you survived the washing machine of life. It's the courage to keep going that matters and you've proven you've got what it takes.

- Look back at your younger self and give thanks for everything she gave you. Bring her into your joy now.

Chapter Sixteen

Go for It ...

*N*o matter what happened yesterday or what is happening today or what might happen tomorrow, you are an incredible human. Look at all the experience you have. Through your losses and wins, joy and sadness, you are still here. We have faced many difficulties. Some we may share, some we shall never share. Times when we thought we'd never get out of bed again … and yet … we did.

I look back and see that there was always something in me that got me through. Sheer bloody-mindedness? A desire to survive? An inherited courage that got my relatives through their own crises? Heaven only knows. But I did manage to unearth in myself a core of resilience which made me think about Repowering as a concept. It gave me a fresh perspective on how you, I and everyone can choose to reframe their life. It is up to us and only us to reach back into the person we used to be. The one who was excited about every party, meeting new friends, finding our talents and using them well. I can either worry about the years ahead – the unknown illnesses, loneliness and setbacks – or I can choose to focus on the real possibility that the future holds fun and joy and new experiences. What would any of us gain by being afraid of the future? Some of it will be a bit scary but why waste your hard-earned power on the negatives? Treat them with respect, yes, but do not worship them forsaking all else.

Am I being a bit Pollyanna-ish? Unfailingly optimistic in the face of adversity, just like the character in the children's book, which was written more than a century ago? While that's the face I try to present to the world, I don't always find life easy. But I have found Repowering to be a great hook to hang my hat on. It pushes me forward and my experience of life tells me there is better stuff to come.

I didn't know it at the time, as I didn't have a word for it then, but I've Repowered several times in my life and from a number of different places. Leaving home in my teens was me taking back my power from my stepfather. When I changed career from theatre to TV, I Repowered myself with the confidence to say, *I can do this.* When I was at the bottom of the dark pit of postnatal depression, I had to do it again, which led to my first divorce and the extra faith I had in building a new life as a single mother.

Leaving *This Morning* was a huge hurdle for me. I loved the show so much, but I was running on empty, so I leapt into an unknown future. I had no idea what would turn up or how I was going to earn a living and then fate presented me with the opportunity to start a writing career. Terrified as I was, I put my fears aside and relied heavily on my internal engine to Repower me.

All these experiences were hard. All of them taught me big lessons. Perhaps the biggest of these was that I can do it.

This time round – exhausted from the pandemic, bereaved of my parents and coming to terms with the end of my marriage – it wasn't easy. But I knew I had the internal reserves that would enable me to survive these mighty earthquake tremors. It took a lot and I'm still on my Repowering journey. If I hadn't started this one when I did, I think I'd still be sitting in tracksuit pants, smoking, drinking and eating too much. Whiling away the time in indolence, achieving nothing.

My 'Era of Indolence' I see as being a field left fallow. I had produced so much that I was exhausted of anything good. I wanted to be fruitful and energised but I had to rest first. I needed to permit myself some leeway and have a break from the world before I was able to come back ready to take on anything.

Everyone can point to testing times they've endured, and I'm no different. I've met with dilemmas that have hurt me and I have had to dig deep to survive. Having good people who hear you and offer the right advice and comfort is excellent fuel for Repowering. And there are so many types of friends. Some stay for life, others for a chapter or even a short paragraph. However a friendship starts or ends, it was always meant to be that way. Never force something that was not going to last. It's nobody's fault.

In many ways my life has panned out in a way I hadn't expected. I never imagined myself to be blessed with four children, two husbands, a dream job and now a career in writing. I wasn't expecting to find myself single, in a tiny and tranquil Cornish village with new friends and laughter. But what joy this new and simple life is bringing me. My social life is small but warm; I do not need much entertaining to keep my spirits up. Church and a weekly line-dancing class are my 'going out out' pleasures.

Since I was 22, I have worked in the public eye. Some people may like me, some people may not. It's a fact of life and one that I accept. I suppose people have a view of who I am, maybe far from the real me. In truth, I'm quite shy. I like simple. I like quiet. I like my own company. I love my friends and I love staying in. It takes a lot to winkle me out of the house!

My life now is peaceful and perhaps a little dull ... just as I like it. Of course, I have down days and sometimes find it difficult to feel I have total control over my life. But, like every single one of us, I am a work in progress.

One thing I never regret though is taking back my power. It has enabled me to create the world I have always wanted. It's not perfect. Nothing is. It's not without pain or worry. None of us get a life that easy. But it is mine and now I can even entertain the thought that maybe I can be proud of the things I have achieved and forgive myself for things I messed up.

Who knows what is around the corner? Seize the day and tackle it right now. You are not alone. There are many of us who are just like you. Women in our forties, fifties, sixties, seventies and beyond. We must reconnect with the young and energetic women we were before we so profligately spent our power on others.

We are taking back our power and creating beautiful, vibrant and interesting lives.

We have the power to Repower now.

Go for it!

Acknowledgements

Not so long ago, somewhere over the past 50 years, I realised that I had been losing the energy, optimism and enthusiasm I had in my teens and early twenties. Back then, my life was free of any anchor of responsibility. Until I had to grow up and attend with respect to my work, my mortgage, marriage and motherhood. That part of my life was exceptionally fulfilling and happy and for most of it I still perceived myself as young. Then one day I lost touch with that self-perception and began to hear the sands of time running out. That's when the word Repowering came to me. It embodied a way for all of us in our sixties to reach back and connect with the person who is still very much within us. You might have been a heller (a lovely Cornish word for a troublemaker) in your younger life, in trouble with yourself and others, but the you who got you out of there is ready to give you a good kick up the backside today.

I want to thank my editor at Ebury Spotlight, the kindest, most patient and thoughtful person, Michelle Warner. We met on Zoom and she absolutely 'got' the whole concept of Repowering. I also want to thank Laura James and Karen Farrington, who helped to knock the manuscript into a sensible shape. As ever, my thanks to Luigi Bonomi, uber literary agent and the man who unwittingly set my mind to thinking about Repowering. He and John Rush guide me and keep the faith whenever I wobble.

And finally, my thanks to you for picking this book up. Let me know your thoughts.

All my love

Fern xx